student study
ART NOTEBOOK

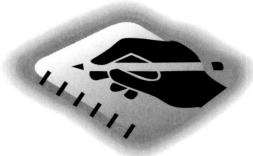

D1710732

ANATOMY

&

physiology

fourth edition

Kent M. Van De Graaff

Stuart Ira Fox

Concepts of

HUMAN

WCB
Wm. C. Brown Publishers
Dubuque, IA Bogota Boston Buenos Aires Caracas Chicago
Guilford, CT London Madrid Mexico City Sydney Toronto

Wm. C. Brown Communications, Inc.

President and Chief Executive Officer *G. Franklin Lewis*
Senior Vice President, Operations *James H. Higby*
Corporate Senior Vice President, President of WCB Manufacturing *Roger Meyer*
Corporate Senior Vice President and Chief Financial Officer *Robert Chesterman*

The credits section for this book begins on page 183 and
is considered an extension of the copyright page.

ISBN 0–697–24395–8

Printed in the United States of America by Wm. C. Brown Communications, Inc.,
2460 Kerper Boulevard, Dubuque, IA 52001

10 9 8 7 6 5 4 3 2 1

This Student Study Art Notebook is a gratis ancillary to assist students in note taking during lectures. On each page, there are one, two, or sometimes three figures faithfully reproduced from the textbook. Each figure also corresponds to one of the 200 acetates available to instructors who adopt this textbook.

The intention is to place the acetate art in front of students (via the notebook) as the instructor uses the overhead during lectures. The advantage to the student is that he/she will be able to see all labels clearly, and take meaningful notes without having to make hurried sketches of the acetate figure.

The pages of the Art Notebook are perforated and three-hole punched, so they can be removed and placed in a personal binder for specific study and review, or to create space for additional notes.

DIRECTORY OF NOTEBOOK FIGURES

TO ACCOMPANY

KENT M. VAN DE GRAAFF AND STUART IRA FOX

CONCEPTS OF HUMAN ANATOMY AND PHYSIOLOGY, 4/E

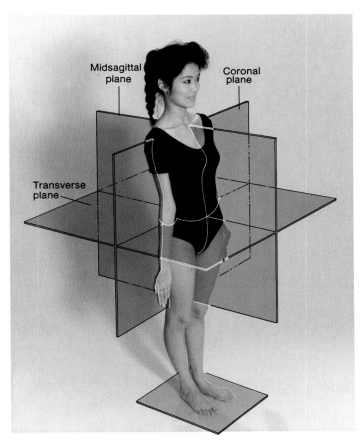

Planes of Reference
Figure 1.11

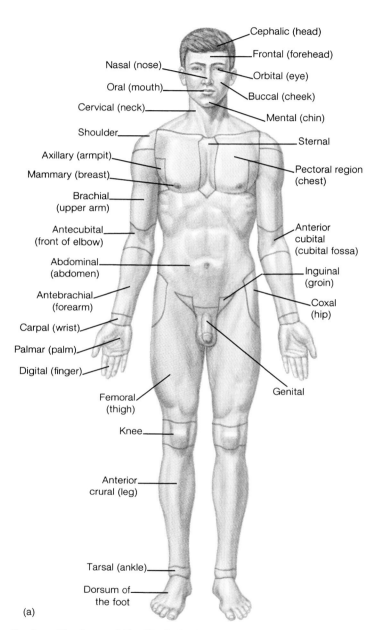

Cephalic (head)
Frontal (forehead)
Nasal (nose)
Orbital (eye)
Oral (mouth)
Buccal (cheek)
Cervical (neck)
Mental (chin)
Shoulder
Sternal
Axillary (armpit)
Mammary (breast)
Pectoral region (chest)
Brachial (upper arm)
Antecubital (front of elbow)
Anterior cubital (cubital fossa)
Abdominal (abdomen)
Inguinal (groin)
Antebrachial (forearm)
Coxal (hip)
Carpal (wrist)
Palmar (palm)
Digital (finger)
Genital
Femoral (thigh)
Knee
Anterior crural (leg)
Tarsal (ankle)
Dorsum of the foot

(a)

Surface Regions of the Body in Anterior View
Figure 1.13a

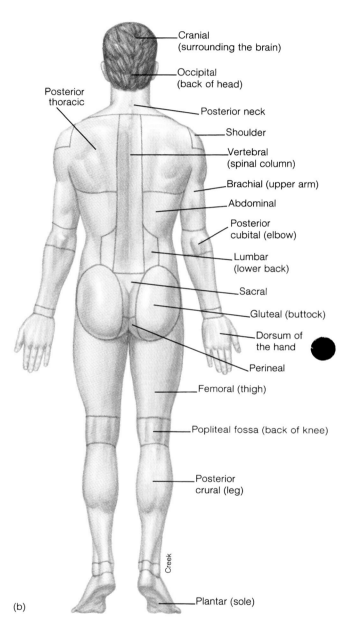

Cranial (surrounding the brain)
Occipital (back of head)
Posterior thoracic
Posterior neck
Shoulder
Vertebral (spinal column)
Brachial (upper arm)
Abdominal
Posterior cubital (elbow)
Lumbar (lower back)
Sacral
Gluteal (buttock)
Dorsum of the hand
Perineal
Femoral (thigh)
Popliteal fossa (back of knee)
Posterior crural (leg)
Creek
Plantar (sole)

(b)

Surface Regions of the Body in Posterior View
Figure 1.13b

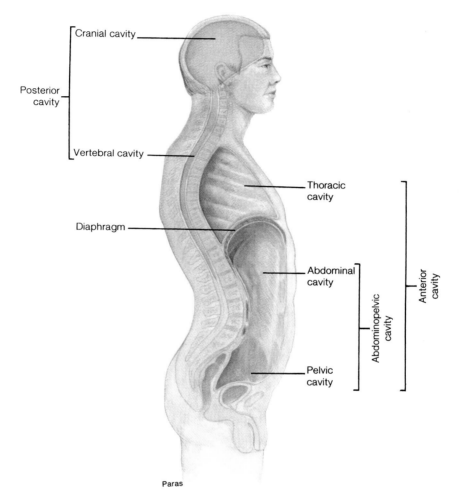

Cranial cavity

Posterior cavity

Vertebral cavity

Thoracic cavity

Diaphragm

Abdominal cavity

Abdominopelvic cavity

Anterior cavity

Pelvic cavity

Paras

Body Cavities
Figure 1.15

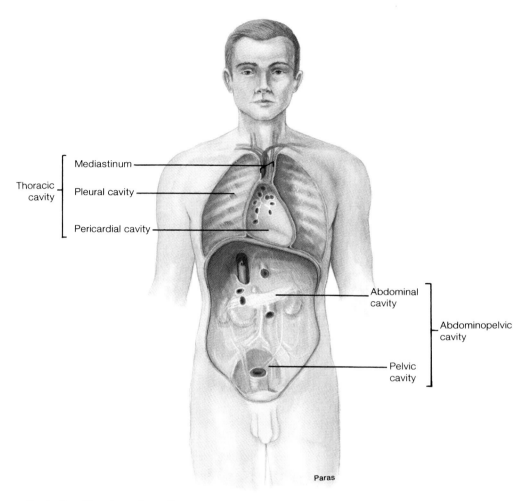

Thoracic cavity
- Mediastinum
- Pleural cavity
- Pericardial cavity

Abdominopelvic cavity
- Abdominal cavity
- Pelvic cavity

Paras

Body Cavities (*continued*)
Figure 1.16

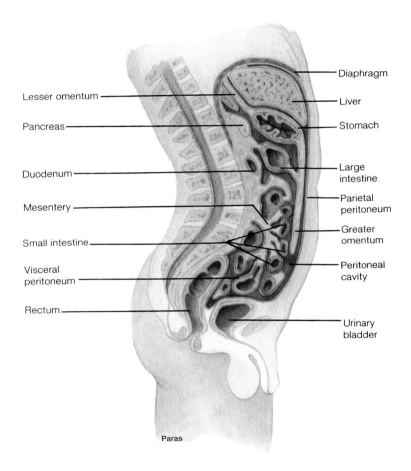

Lesser omentum

Pancreas

Duodenum

Mesentery

Small intestine

Visceral peritoneum

Rectum

Diaphragm

Liver

Stomach

Large intestine

Parietal peritoneum

Greater omentum

Peritoneal cavity

Urinary bladder

Paras

Visceral Organs and Serous Membranes
Figure 1.17

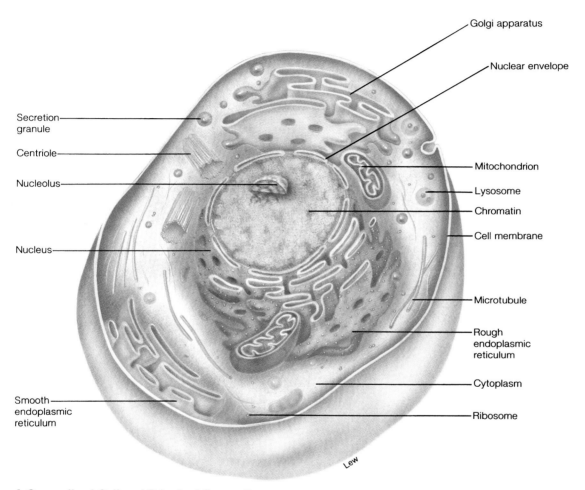

Golgi apparatus

Nuclear envelope

Secretion
granule

Centriole

Nucleolus

Nucleus

Smooth
endoplasmic
reticulum

Mitochondrion

Lysosome

Chromatin

Cell membrane

Microtubule

Rough
endoplasmic
reticulum

Cytoplasm

Ribosome

Lew

A Generalized Cell and Principal Organelles
Figure 3.1

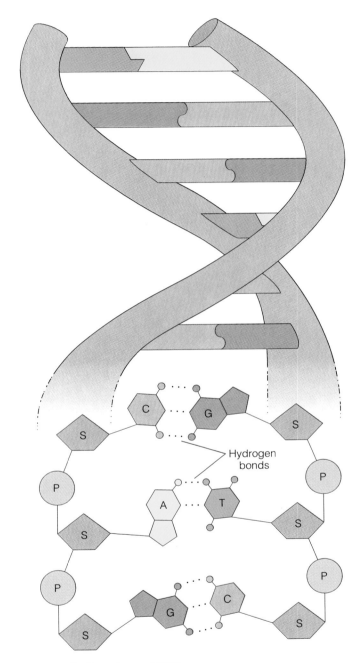

Double Helix Structure of DNA
Figure 3.16

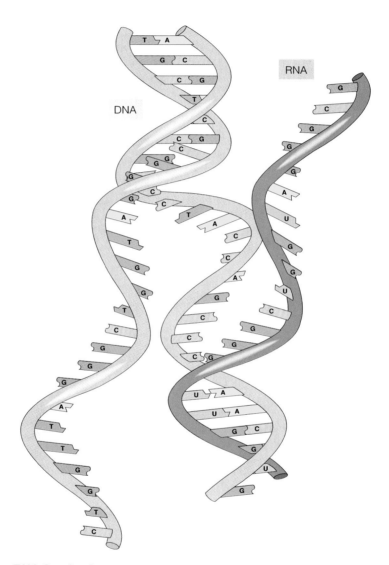

DNA

RNA

RNA Synthesis
Figure 3.19

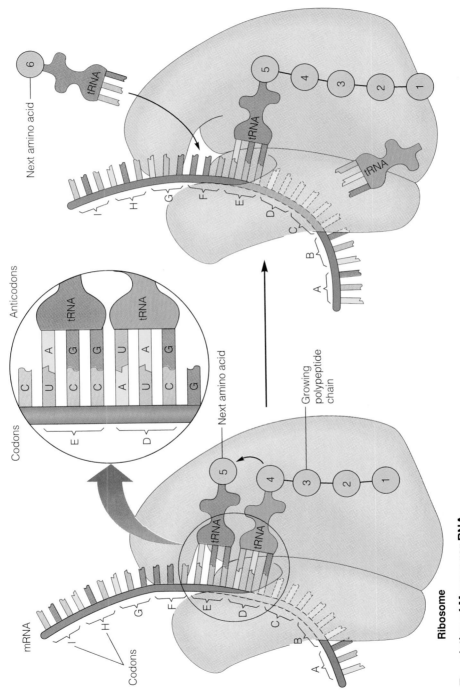

Next amino acid

Anticodons

Codons

E			D		
C	U	C	C	A	U
A	G	C	G	U	A
					G

tRNA

tRNA

Codons

Next amino acid

Growing
polypeptide
chain

mRNA

Ribosome

Translation of Messenger RNA
Figure 3.23

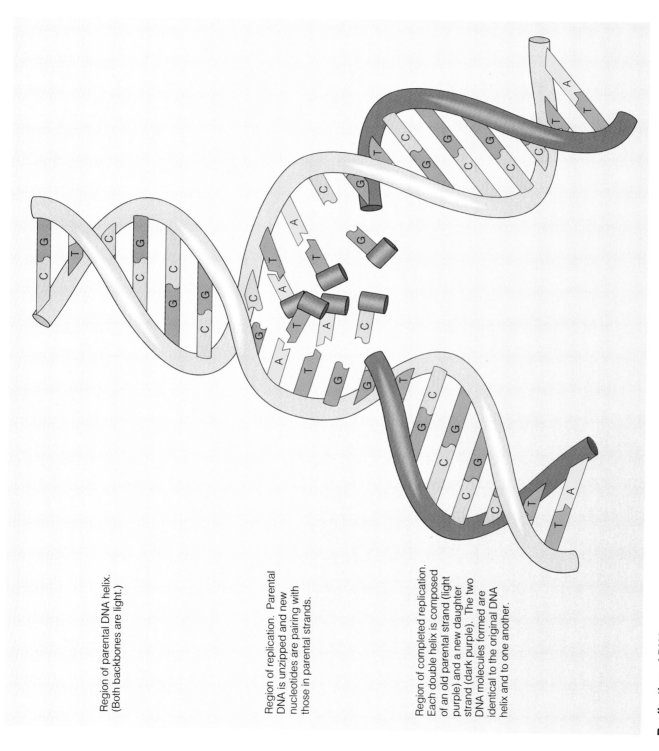

Region of parental DNA helix. (Both backbones are light.)

Region of replication. Parental DNA is unzipped and new nucleotides are pairing with those in parental strands.

Region of completed replication. Each double helix is composed of an old parental strand (light purple) and a new daughter strand (dark purple). The two DNA molecules formed are identical to the original DNA helix and to one another.

Replication of DNA
Figure 3.26

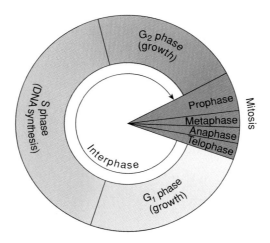

Life Cycle of a Cell
Figure 3.27

(a) Interphase

- The chromosomes are in an extended form and seen as chromatin in the electron microscope.
- The nucleus is visible.

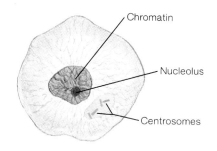
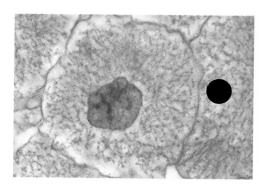

(b) Prophase

- The chromosomes are seen to consist of two chromatids joined by a centromere.
- The centrioles move apart toward opposite poles of the cell.
- Spindle fibers are produced and extended from each centrosome.
- The nuclear membrane starts to disappear.
- The nucleolus is no longer visible.

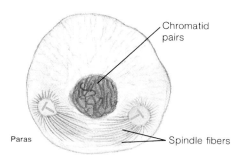
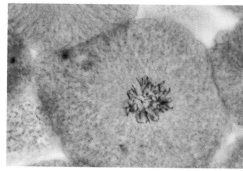

(c) Metaphase

- The chromosomes are lined up at the equator of the cell.
- The spindle fibers from each centriole are attached to the centromeres of the chromosomes.
- The nuclear membrane has disappeared.

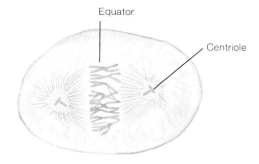
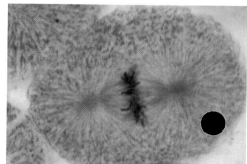

(d) Anaphase

- The centromeres split, and the sister chromatids separate as each is pulled to an opposite pole.

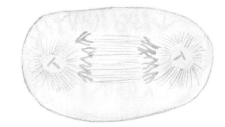
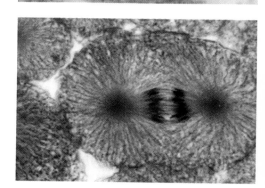

(e) Telophase

- The chromosomes become longer, thinner, and less distance.
- New nuclear membranes form.
- The nucleolus reappears.
- Cell division is nearly complete.

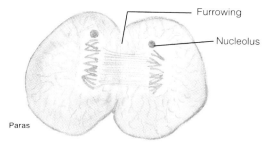
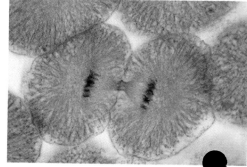

Stages of Mitosis
Figure 3.30a–e

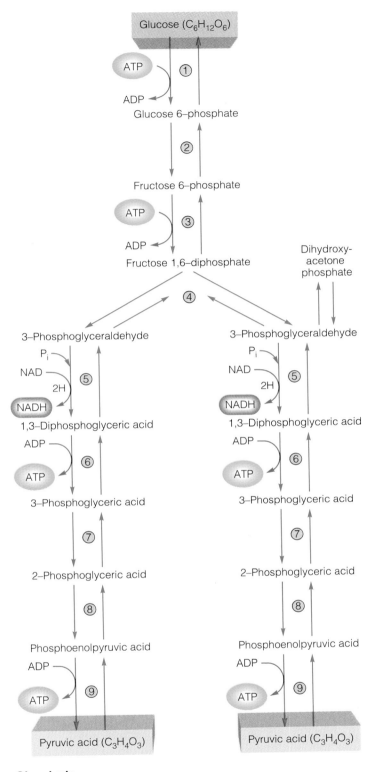

Glycolysis
Figure 4.18

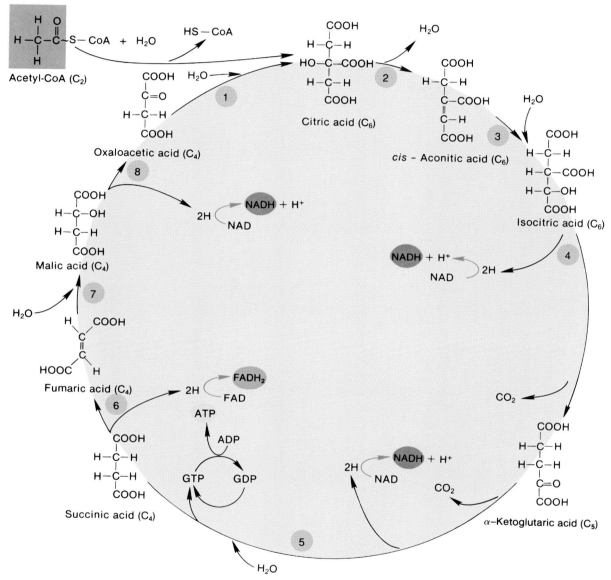

Krebs Cycle
Figure 4.23

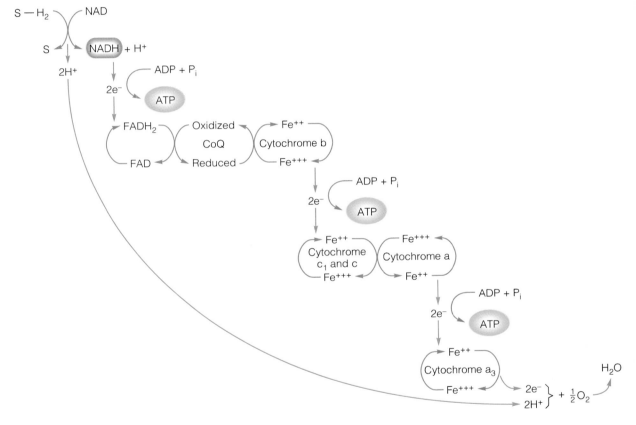

Electron Transport and Oxidative Phosphorylation
Figure 4.24

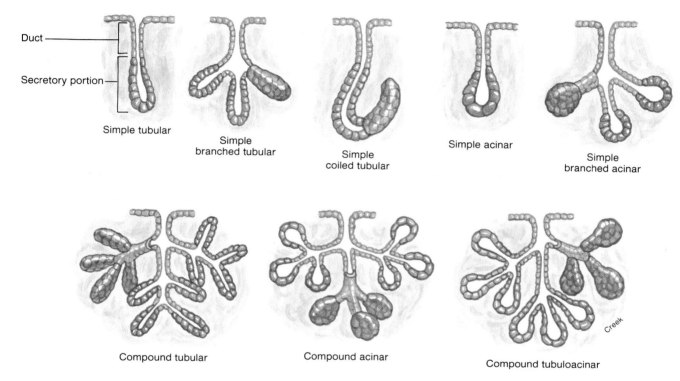

Duct

Secretory portion

Simple tubular

Simple
branched tubular

Simple
coiled tubular

Simple acinar

Simple
branched acinar

Compound tubular

Compound acinar

Compound tubuloacinar

Creek

Multicellular Exocrine Glands
Figure 6.12

Table 7.2 Layers of the epidermis

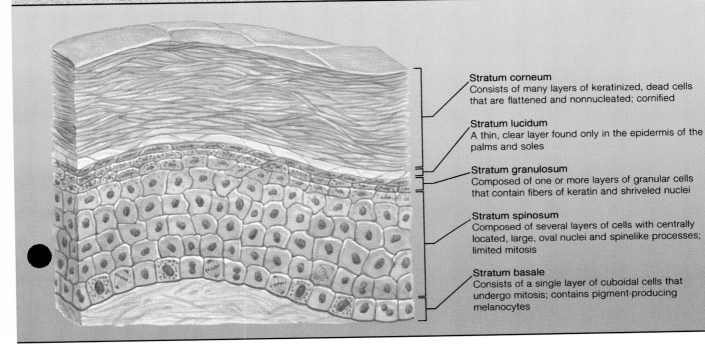

Stratum corneum
Consists of many layers of keratinized, dead cells that are flattened and nonnucleated; cornified

Stratum lucidum
A thin, clear layer found only in the epidermis of the palms and soles

Stratum granulosum
Composed of one or more layers of granular cells that contain fibers of keratin and shriveled nuclei

Stratum spinosum
Composed of several layers of cells with centrally located, large, oval nuclei and spinelike processes; limited mitosis

Stratum basale
Consists of a single layer of cuboidal cells that undergo mitosis; contains pigment-producing melanocytes

Layers of Epidermis
Table 7.2

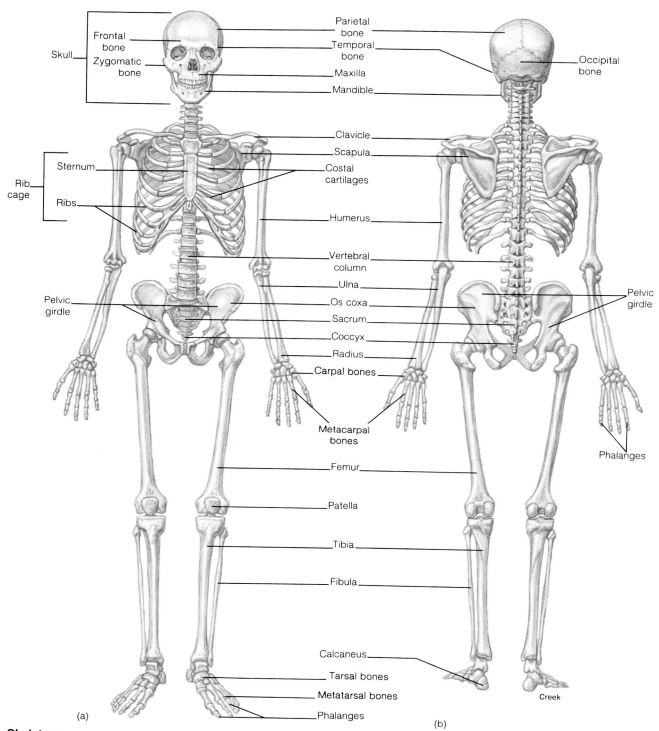

Skull
Frontal bone
Zygomatic bone

Parietal bone
Temporal bone
Maxilla
Mandible

Occipital bone

Clavicle
Scapula
Costal cartilages

Sternum
Rib cage
Ribs

Humerus

Vertebral column
Ulna
Os coxa
Sacrum
Coccyx
Radius
Carpal bones

Pelvic girdle

Pelvic girdle

Metacarpal bones

Phalanges

Femur

Patella

Tibia

Fibula

Calcaneus
Tarsal bones
Metatarsal bones
Phalanges

(a)

(b)

Creek

Skeleton
Figure 8.1

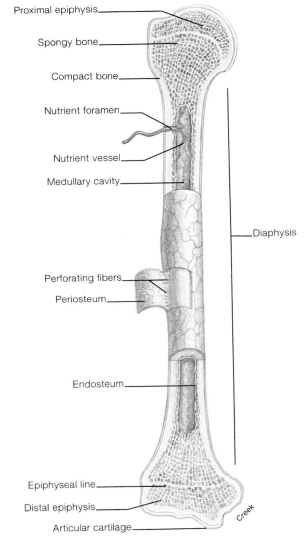

Proximal epiphysis

Spongy bone

Compact bone

Nutrient foramen

Nutrient vessel

Medullary cavity

Diaphysis

Perforating fibers

Periosteum

Endosteum

Epiphyseal line

Distal epiphysis

Articular cartilage

Creek

Structure of a Long Bone
Figure 8.4

19

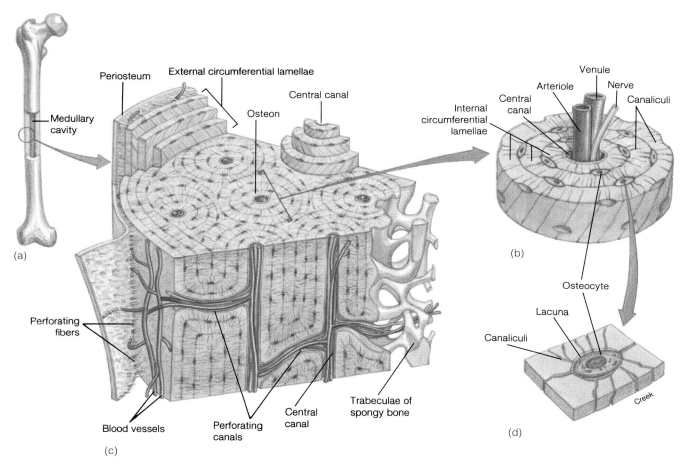

(a)

(c)

(b)

(d)

Labels in figure:
Periosteum
External circumferential lamellae
Central canal
Osteon
Medullary cavity
Venule
Arteriole
Nerve
Canaliculi
Central canal
Internal circumferential lamellae
Perforating fibers
Osteocyte
Lacuna
Canaliculi
Blood vessels
Perforating canals
Central canal
Trabeculae of spongy bone
Creek

Compact Bone Tissue
Figure 8.6

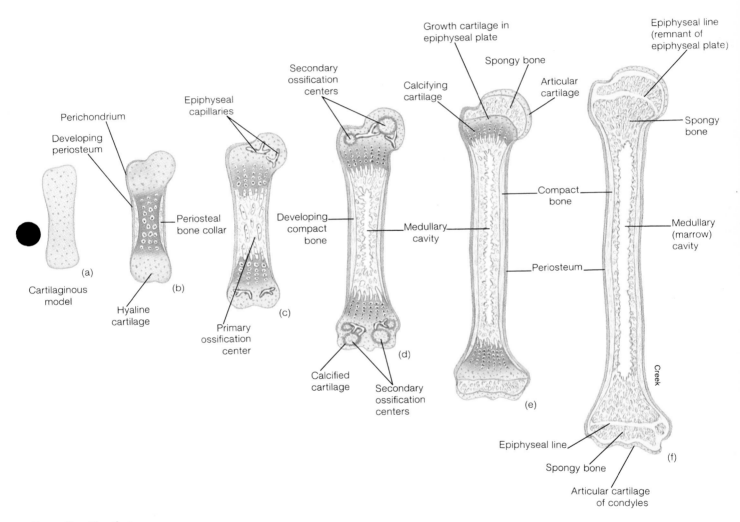

Bone Ossification
Figure 8.9

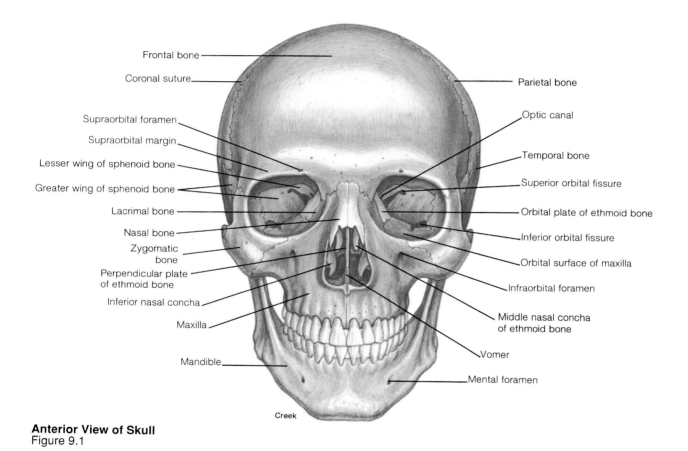

Frontal bone

Coronal suture

Parietal bone

Supraorbital foramen

Supraorbital margin

Optic canal

Lesser wing of sphenoid bone

Temporal bone

Greater wing of sphenoid bone

Superior orbital fissure

Lacrimal bone

Orbital plate of ethmoid bone

Nasal bone

Inferior orbital fissure

Zygomatic bone

Orbital surface of maxilla

Perpendicular plate of ethmoid bone

Infraorbital foramen

Inferior nasal concha

Middle nasal concha of ethmoid bone

Maxilla

Mandible

Vomer

Mental foramen

Creek

Anterior View of Skull
Figure 9.1

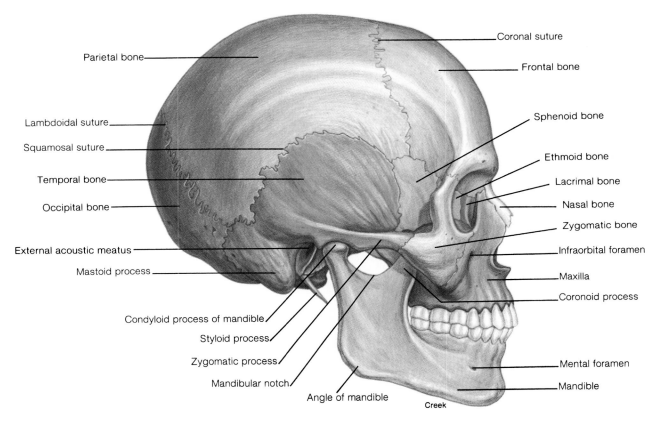

Coronal suture

Parietal bone

Frontal bone

Sphenoid bone

Lambdoidal suture

Squamosal suture

Ethmoid bone

Temporal bone

Lacrimal bone

Occipital bone

Nasal bone

Zygomatic bone

External acoustic meatus

Infraorbital foramen

Mastoid process

Maxilla

Coronoid process

Condyloid process of mandible

Styloid process

Zygomatic process

Mental foramen

Mandibular notch

Mandible

Angle of mandible

Creek

Lateral View of Skull
Figure 9.2

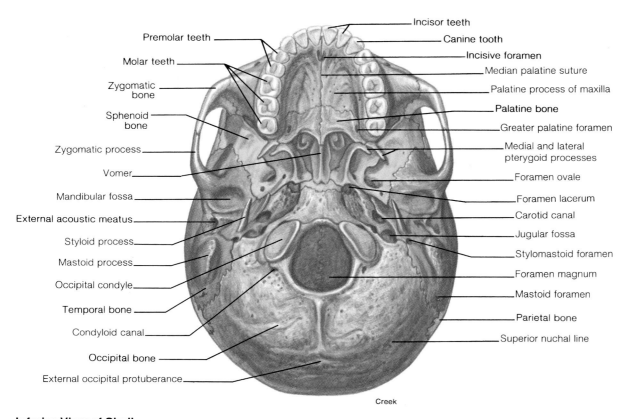

Premolar teeth
Molar teeth
Zygomatic bone
Sphenoid bone
Zygomatic process
Vomer
Mandibular fossa
External acoustic meatus
Styloid process
Mastoid process
Occipital condyle
Temporal bone
Condyloid canal
Occipital bone
External occipital protuberance

Incisor teeth
Canine tooth
Incisive foramen
Median palatine suture
Palatine process of maxilla
Palatine bone
Greater palatine foramen
Medial and lateral pterygoid processes
Foramen ovale
Foramen lacerum
Carotid canal
Jugular fossa
Stylomastoid foramen
Foramen magnum
Mastoid foramen
Parietal bone
Superior nuchal line

Creek

Inferior View of Skull
Figure 9.3

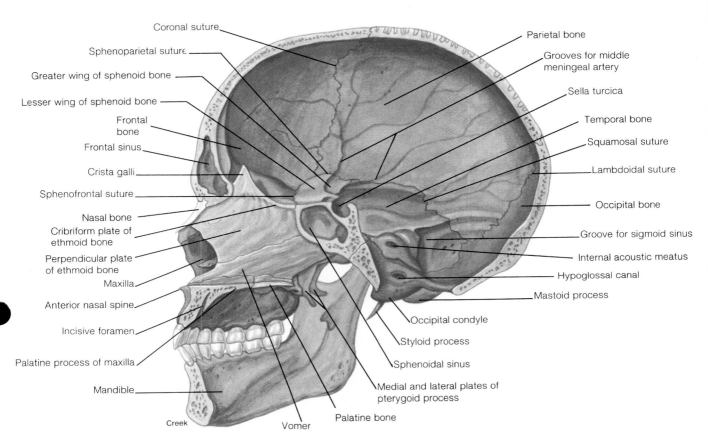

Coronal suture

Sphenoparietal suture

Greater wing of sphenoid bone

Lesser wing of sphenoid bone

Frontal bone

Frontal sinus

Crista galli

Sphenofrontal suture

Nasal bone

Cribriform plate of ethmoid bone

Perpendicular plate of ethmoid bone

Maxilla

Anterior nasal spine

Incisive foramen

Palatine process of maxilla

Mandible

Creek

Parietal bone

Grooves for middle meningeal artery

Sella turcica

Temporal bone

Squamosal suture

Lambdoidal suture

Occipital bone

Groove for sigmoid sinus

Internal acoustic meatus

Hypoglossal canal

Mastoid process

Occipital condyle

Styloid process

Sphenoidal sinus

Medial and lateral plates of pterygoid process

Palatine bone

Vomer

Midsagittal View of Skull
Figure 9.4

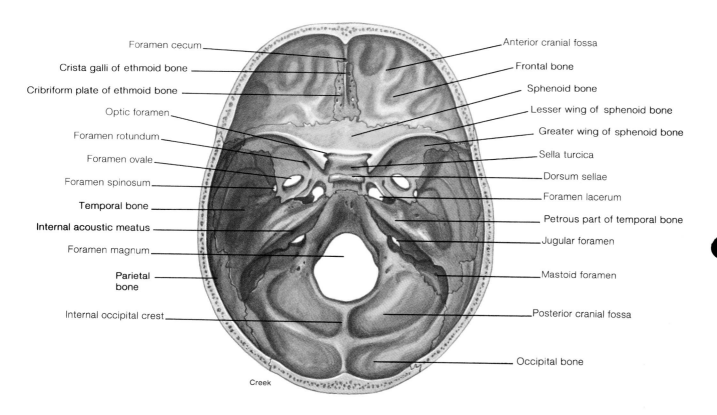

Foramen cecum

Crista galli of ethmoid bone

Cribriform plate of ethmoid bone

Optic foramen

Foramen rotundum

Foramen ovale

Foramen spinosum

Temporal bone

Internal acoustic meatus

Foramen magnum

Parietal bone

Internal occipital crest

Anterior cranial fossa

Frontal bone

Sphenoid bone

Lesser wing of sphenoid bone

Greater wing of sphenoid bone

Sella turcica

Dorsum sellae

Foramen lacerum

Petrous part of temporal bone

Jugular foramen

Mastoid foramen

Posterior cranial fossa

Occipital bone

Creek

Floor of Cranial Cavity
Figure 9.6

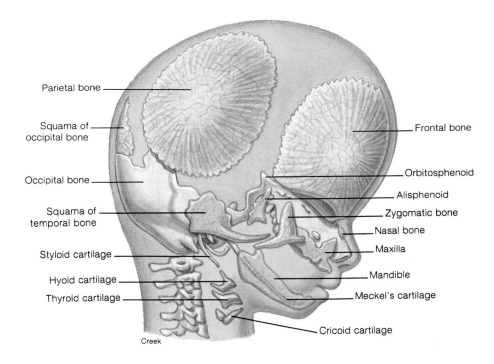

Embryonic Skull at Twelve Weeks
Box Figure 9.1, Figure 1

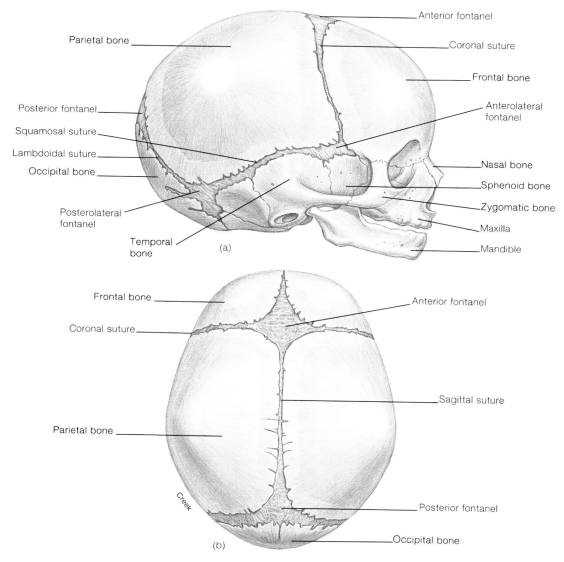

Parietal bone

Anterior fontanel

Coronal suture

Frontal bone

Posterior fontanel

Anterolateral
fontanel

Squamosal suture

Lambdoidal suture

Occipital bone

Nasal bone

Sphenoid bone

Zygomatic bone

Posterolateral
fontanel

Maxilla

Temporal
bone

Mandible

(a)

Frontal bone

Anterior fontanel

Coronal suture

Sagittal suture

Parietal bone

Creek

Posterior fontanel

Occipital bone

(b)

Fetal Skull
Box Figure 9.1, Figure 2

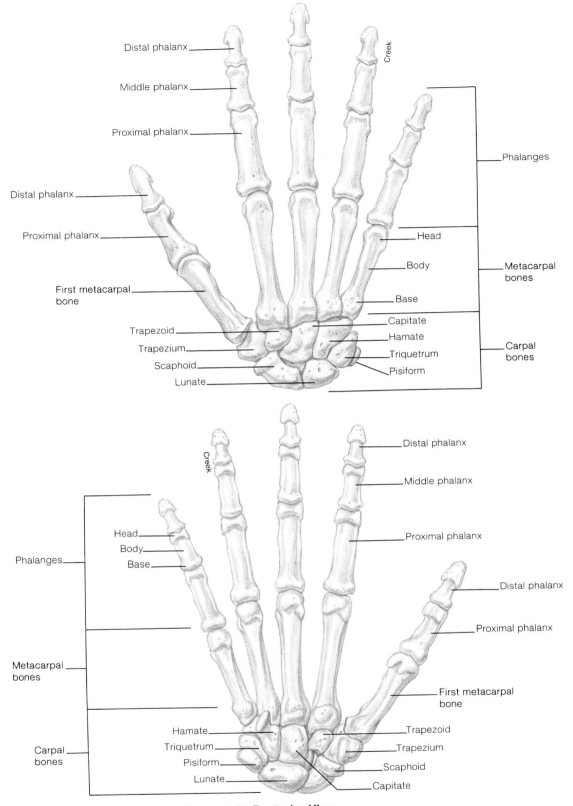

Bones of Hand: (a) Anterior View and (b) Posterior View
Figure 10.7a and 10.8

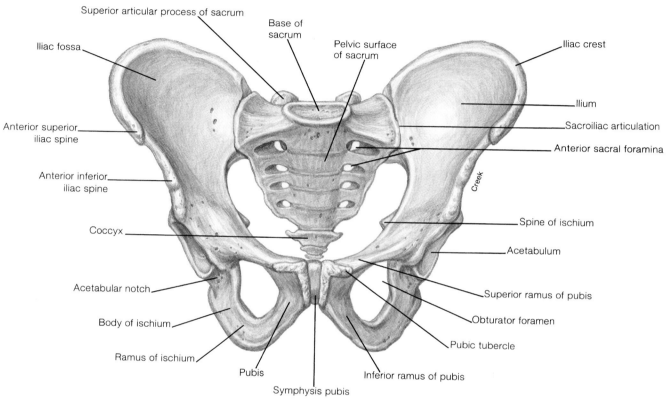

Superior articular process of sacrum

Base of sacrum

Pelvic surface of sacrum

Iliac crest

Iliac fossa

Iliac fossa

Iliac crest

Ilium

Anterior superior iliac spine

Sacroiliac articulation

Anterior sacral foramina

Anterior inferior iliac spine

Coccyx

Spine of ischium

Acetabulum

Acetabular notch

Superior ramus of pubis

Body of ischium

Obturator foramen

Ramus of ischium

Pubic tubercle

Pubis

Inferior ramus of pubis

Symphysis pubis

Creek

Anterior View of Pelvic Girdle
Figure 10.10

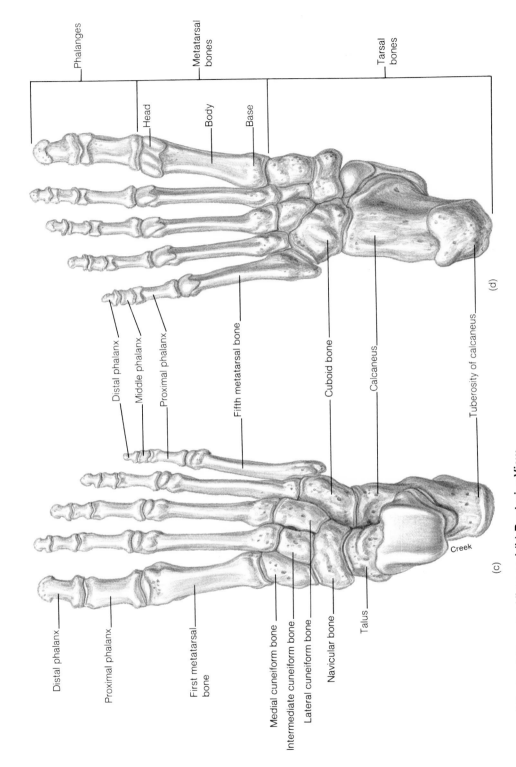

Phalanges

Metatarsal
bones

Tarsal
bones

Head

Body

Base

(d)

Distal phalanx

Middle phalanx

Proximal phalanx

Fifth metatarsal bone

Cuboid bone

Calcaneus

Tuberosity of calcaneus

Distal phalanx

Proximal phalanx

First metatarsal
bone

Medial cuneiform bone

Intermediate cuneiform bone

Lateral cuneiform bone

Navicular bone

Talus

Creek

(c)

Bones of Foot: (a) Superior View and (b) Posterior View
Figure 10.18c,d

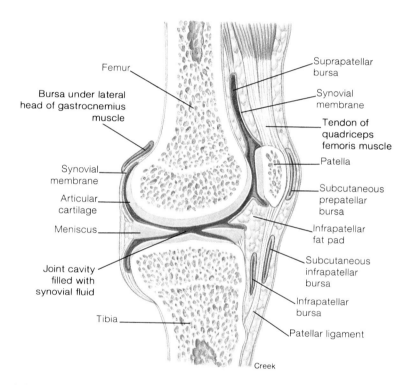

Femur

Bursa under lateral
head of gastrocnemius
muscle

Synovial
membrane

Articular
cartilage

Meniscus

Joint cavity
filled with
synovial fluid

Tibia

Suprapatellar
bursa

Synovial
membrane

Tendon of
quadriceps
femoris muscle

Patella

Subcutaneous
prepatellar
bursa

Infrapatellar
fat pad

Subcutaneous
infrapatellar
bursa

Infrapatellar
bursa

Patellar ligament

Creek

A Synovial Joint
Figure 11.5

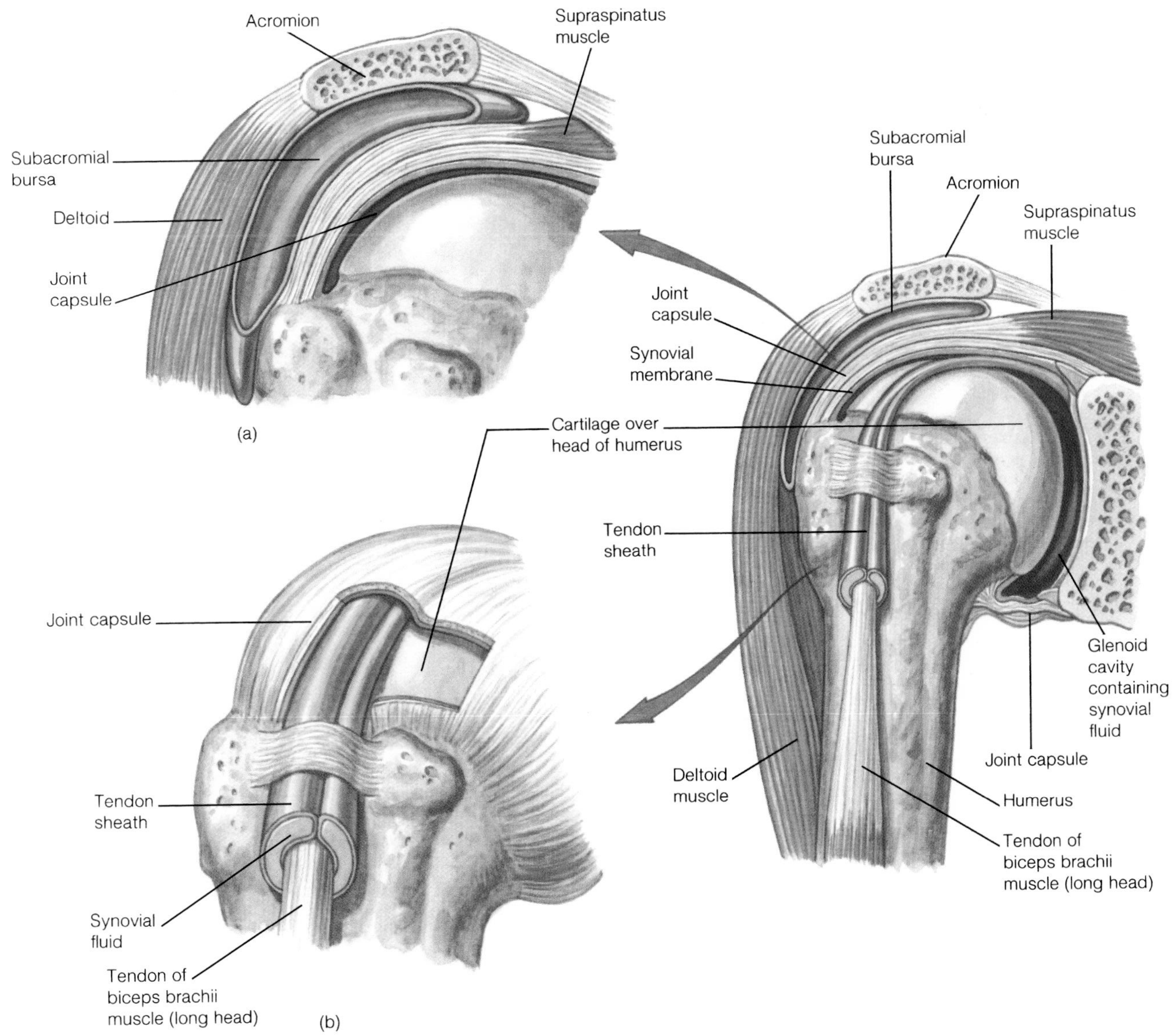

Bursae and Tendon Sheaths
Figure 11.6

Supraspinatus muscle

Acromion

Glenoid cavity containing synovial fluid

Joint capsule

Humerus

Tendon of biceps brachii muscle (long head)

Subacromial bursa

Joint capsule

Synovial membrane

Cartilage over head of humerus

Tendon sheath

Deltoid muscle

Supraspinatus muscle

Acromion

Subacromial bursa

Deltoid

Joint capsule

(a)

Joint capsule

Tendon sheath

Synovial fluid

Tendon of biceps brachii muscle (long head)

(b)

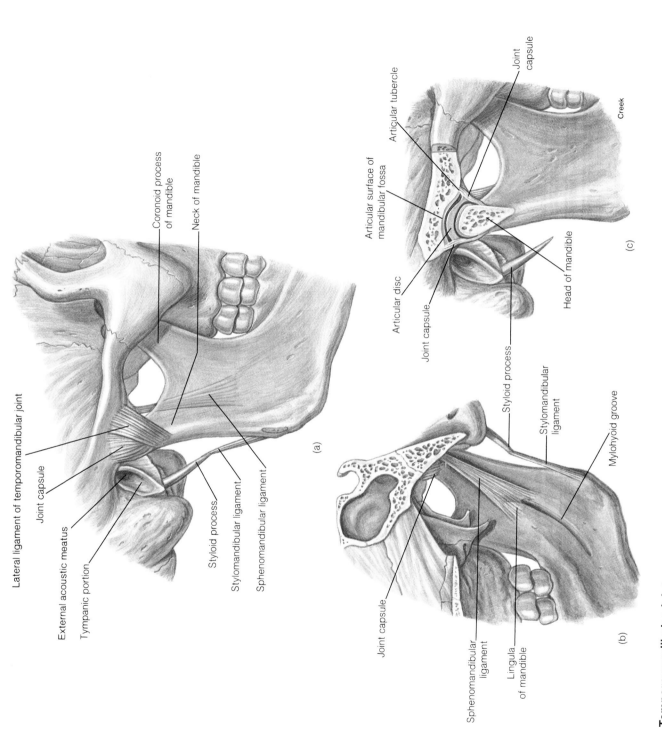

Lateral ligament of temporomandibular joint

Joint capsule

External acoustic meatus

Tympanic portion

Coronoid process of mandible

Neck of mandible

Styloid process

Stylomandibular ligament

Sphenomandibular ligament

(a)

Joint capsule

Sphenomandibular ligament

Lingula of mandible

Styloid process

Stylomandibular ligament

Mylohyoid groove

(b)

Articular tubercle

Joint capsule

Articular surface of mandibular fossa

Articular disc

Joint capsule

Head of mandible

Creek

(c)

Temporomandibular Joint
Figure 11.23

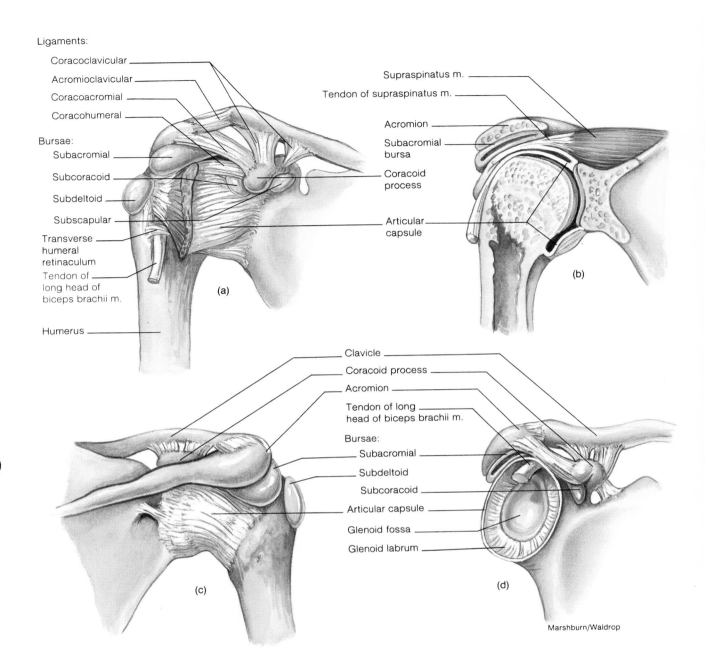

Ligaments:
- Coracoclavicular
- Acromioclavicular
- Coracoacromial
- Coracohumeral

Bursae:
- Subacromial
- Subcoracoid
- Subdeltoid
- Subscapular

Transverse humeral retinaculum

Tendon of long head of biceps brachii m.

Humerus

(a)

Supraspinatus m.
Tendon of supraspinatus m.
Acromion
Subacromial bursa
Coracoid process
Articular capsule

(b)

Clavicle
Coracoid process
Acromion
Tendon of long head of biceps brachii m.

Bursae:
- Subacromial
- Subdeltoid
- Subcoracoid

Articular capsule
Glenoid fossa
Glenoid labrum

(c)

(d)

Marshburn/Waldrop

Humeral (Shoulder) Joint
Figure 11.24

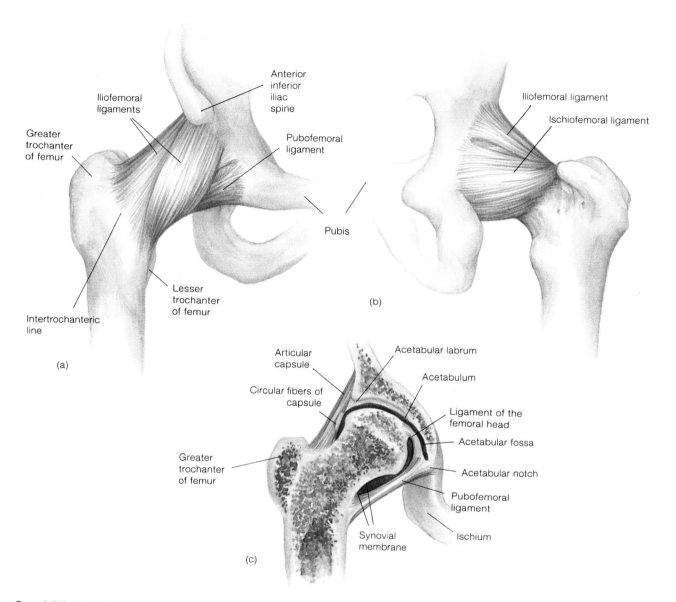

Iliofemoral ligaments

Anterior inferior iliac spine

Greater trochanter of femur

Pubofemoral ligament

Lesser trochanter of femur

Intertrochanteric line

Pubis

(a)

Iliofemoral ligament

Ischiofemoral ligament

(b)

Articular capsule

Acetabular labrum

Acetabulum

Circular fibers of capsule

Ligament of the femoral head

Greater trochanter of femur

Acetabular fossa

Acetabular notch

Pubofemoral ligament

Ischium

Synovial membrane

(c)

Coxal (Hip) Joint
Figure 11.27

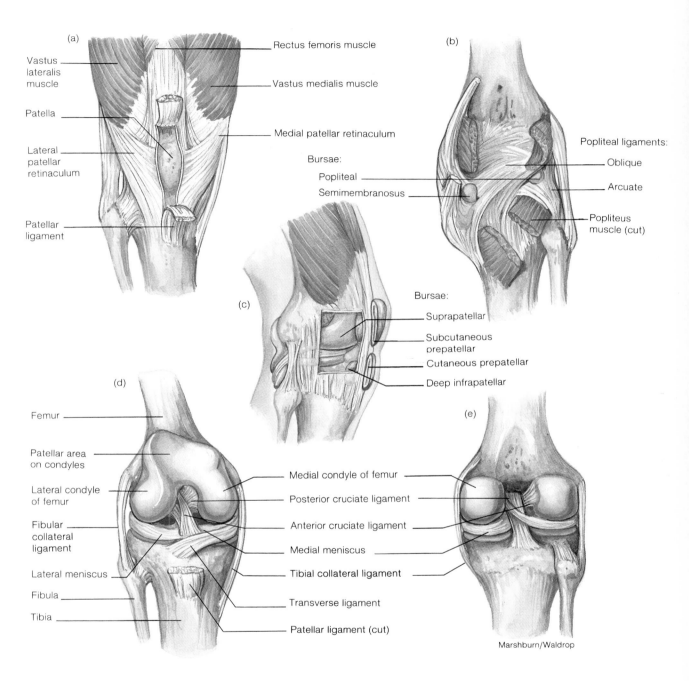

(a)
Vastus lateralis muscle
Patella
Lateral patellar retinaculum
Patellar ligament
Rectus femoris muscle
Vastus medialis muscle
Medial patellar retinaculum

(b)
Bursae:
Popliteal
Semimembranosus
Popliteal ligaments:
Oblique
Arcuate
Popliteus muscle (cut)

(c)
Bursae:
Suprapatellar
Subcutaneous prepatellar
Cutaneous prepatellar
Deep infrapatellar

(d)
Femur
Patellar area on condyles
Lateral condyle of femur
Fibular collateral ligament
Lateral meniscus
Fibula
Tibia
Medial condyle of femur
Posterior cruciate ligament
Anterior cruciate ligament
Medial meniscus
Tibial collateral ligament
Transverse ligament
Patellar ligament (cut)

(e)

Marshburn/Waldrop

Tibiofemoral (Knee) Joint
Figure 11.28

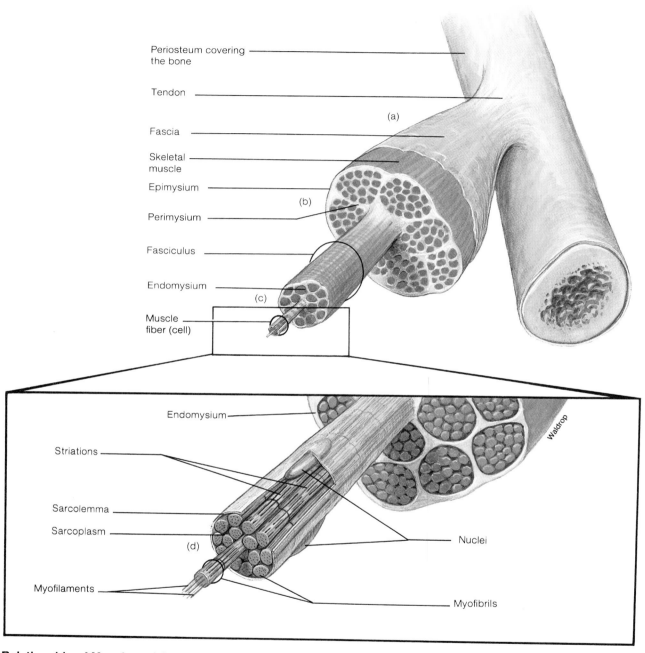

Periosteum covering
the bone

Tendon

(a)

Fascia

Skeletal
muscle

Epimysium

(b)

Perimysium

Fasciculus

Endomysium

(c)

Muscle
fiber (cell)

Waldrop

Endomysium

Striations

Sarcolemma

Sarcoplasm

(d)

Nuclei

Myofilaments

Myofibrils

Relationship of Muscle and Connective Tissue
Figure 12.1

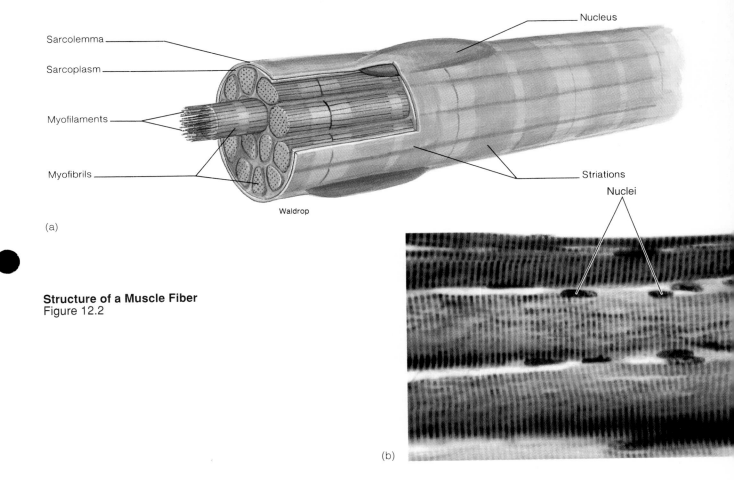

Sarcolemma

Sarcoplasm

Myofilaments

Myofibrils

Waldrop

Nucleus

Striations

Nuclei

(a)

(b)

Structure of a Muscle Fiber
Figure 12.2

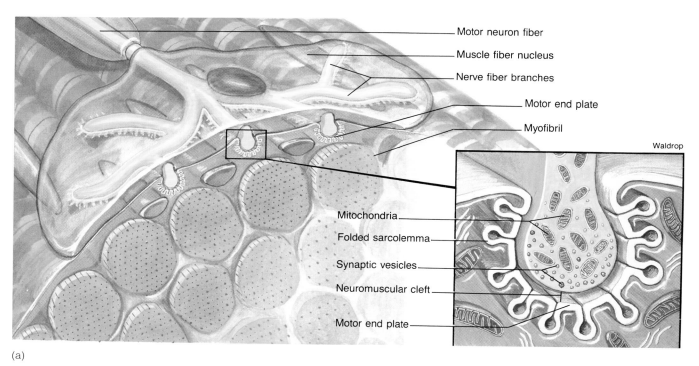

Motor neuron fiber

Muscle fiber nucleus

Nerve fiber branches

Motor end plate

Myofibril

Waldrop

Mitochondria

Folded sarcolemma

Synaptic vesicles

Neuromuscular cleft

Motor end plate

(a)

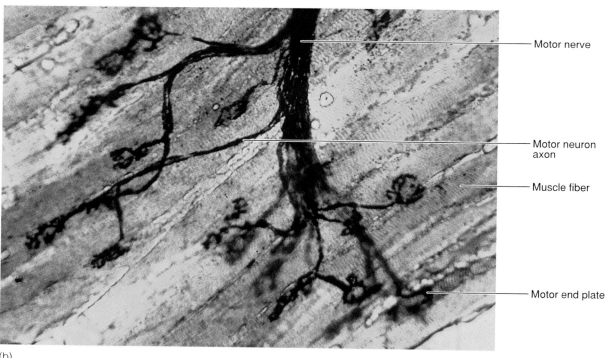

Motor nerve

Motor neuron axon

Muscle fiber

Motor end plate

(b)

Motor End Plate at the Neuromuscular Junction
Figure 12.5

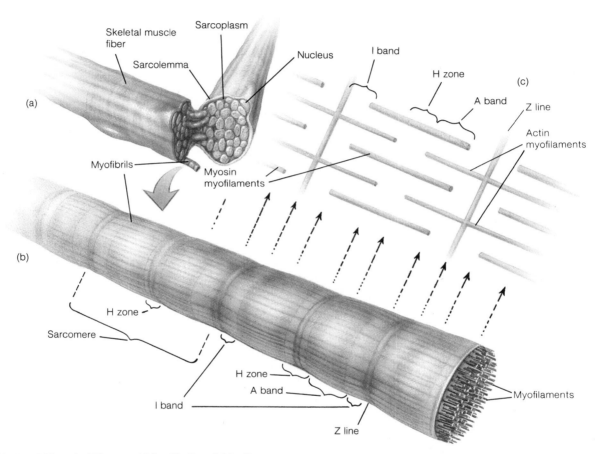

Skeletal Muscle Fiber and Myofibrils within Sarcomeres
Figure 12.7

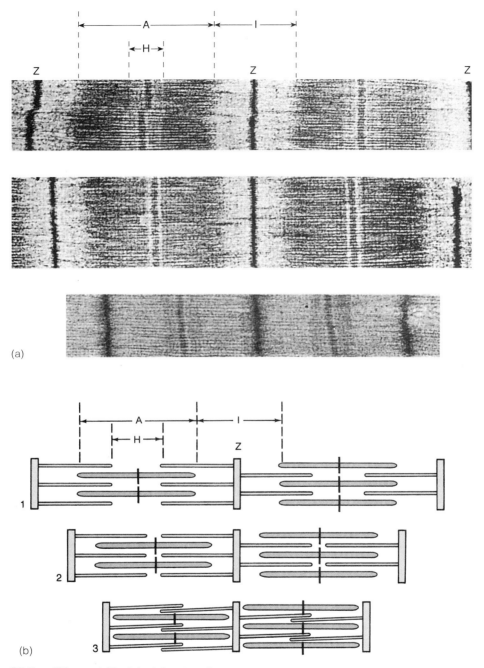

Sliding Filament Model of Contraction
Figure 12.10

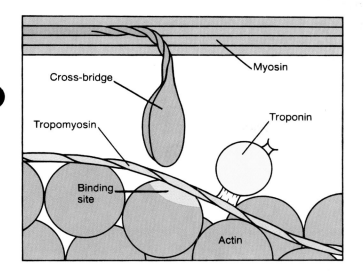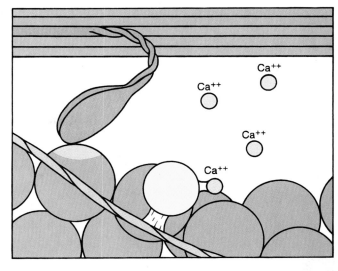

The Effect of Ca⁺⁺ on Myosin Cross-Bridge Attachment to Actin
Figure 12.15

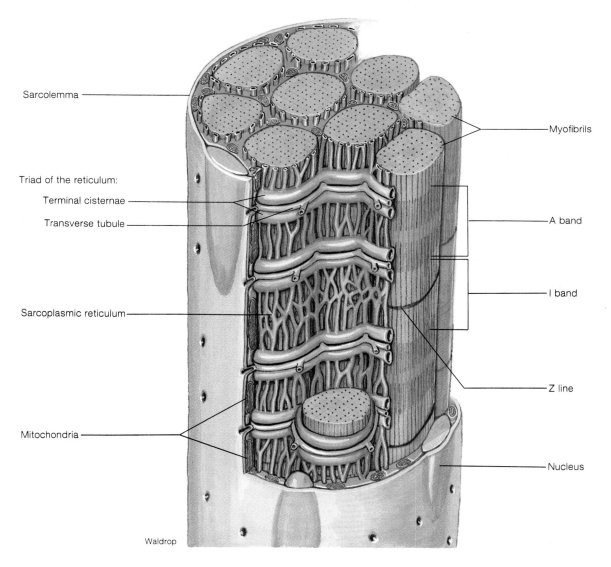

Relationship of Myofibrils and Sarcolemma
Figure 12.16

43

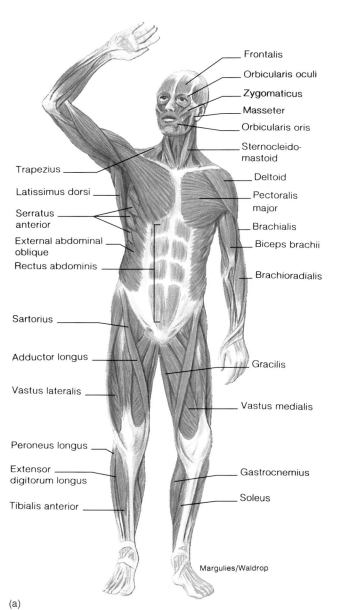

Frontalis
Orbicularis oculi
Zygomaticus
Masseter
Orbicularis oris
Sternocleido-mastoid
Trapezius
Latissimus dorsi
Serratus anterior
External abdominal oblique
Rectus abdominis
Deltoid
Pectoralis major
Brachialis
Biceps brachii
Brachioradialis
Sartorius
Adductor longus
Vastus lateralis
Gracilis
Vastus medialis
Peroneus longus
Extensor digitorum longus
Tibialis anterior
Gastrocnemius
Soleus

Margulies/Waldrop

(a)

Superficial Muscles, Anterior View
Figure 13.1a

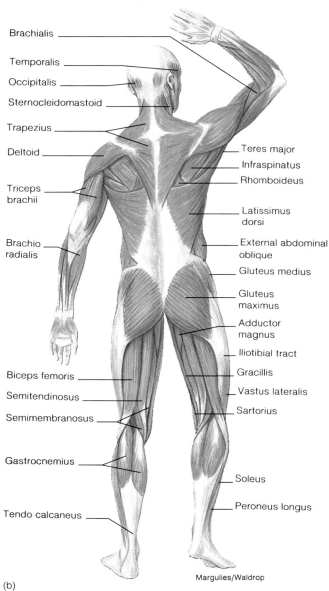

Brachialis
Temporalis
Occipitalis
Sternocleidomastoid
Trapezius
Deltoid
Triceps brachii
Brachio radialis
Teres major
Infraspinatus
Rhomboideus
Latissimus dorsi
External abdominal oblique
Gluteus medius
Gluteus maximus
Adductor magnus
Iliotibial tract
Gracillis
Vastus lateralis
Sartorius
Biceps femoris
Semitendinosus
Semimembranosus
Gastrocnemius
Soleus
Peroneus longus
Tendo calcaneus

Margulies/Waldrop

(b)

Superficial Muscles, Posterior View
Figure 13.1b

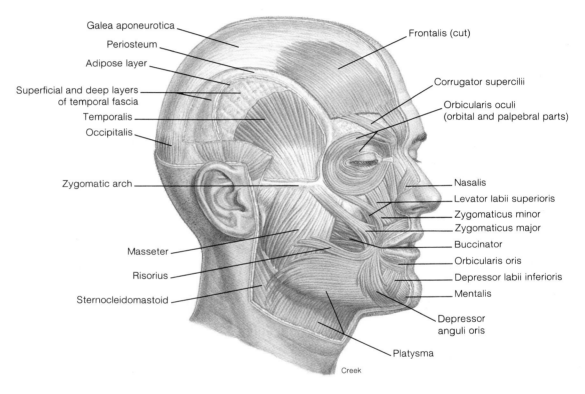

Galea aponeurotica
Periosteum
Adipose layer
Superficial and deep layers of temporal fascia
Temporalis
Occipitalis
Zygomatic arch
Masseter
Risorius
Sternocleidomastoid

Frontalis (cut)
Corrugator supercilii
Orbicularis oculi (orbital and palpebral parts)
Nasalis
Levator labii superioris
Zygomaticus minor
Zygomaticus major
Buccinator
Orbicularis oris
Depressor labii inferioris
Mentalis
Depressor anguli oris
Platysma

Creek

Muscles of Facial Expression
Figure 13.5

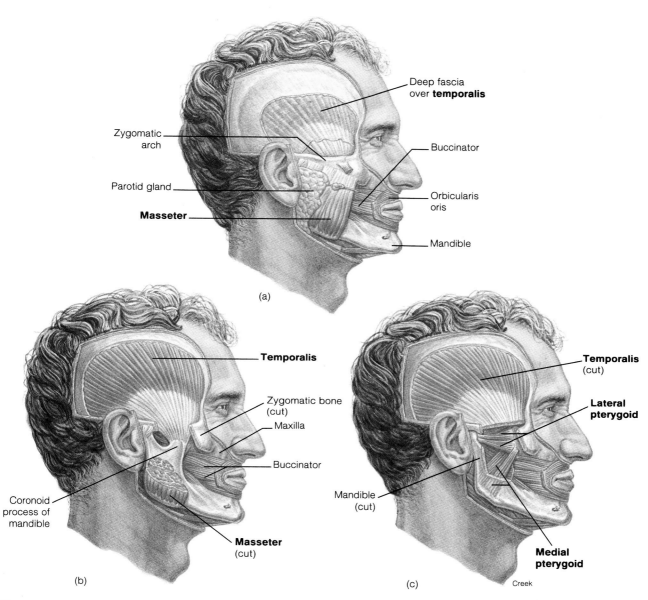

(a)

Deep fascia over **temporalis**

Zygomatic arch

Buccinator

Parotid gland

Orbicularis oris

Masseter

Mandible

Temporalis

Zygomatic bone (cut)

Maxilla

Buccinator

Coronoid process of mandible

Masseter (cut)

(b)

Temporalis (cut)

Lateral pterygoid

Mandible (cut)

Medial pterygoid

(c)

Creek

Muscles of Mastication
Figure 13.6

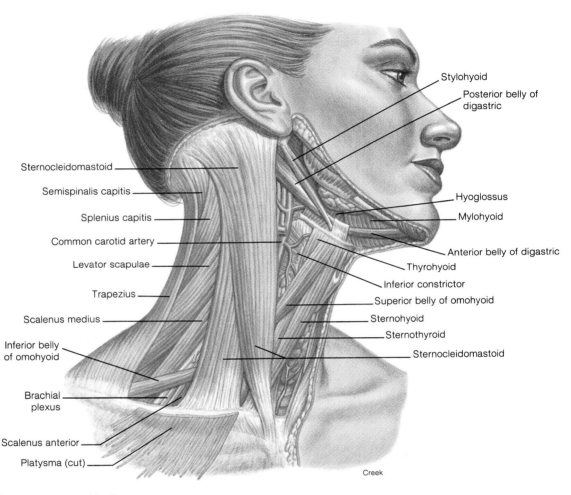

Stylohyoid

Posterior belly of
digastric

Sternocleidomastoid

Semispinalis capitis

Splenius capitis

Common carotid artery

Levator scapulae

Trapezius

Scalenus medius

Inferior belly
of omohyoid

Brachial
plexus

Scalenus anterior

Platysma (cut)

Hyoglossus

Mylohyoid

Anterior belly of digastric

Thyrohyoid

Inferior constrictor

Superior belly of omohyoid

Sternohyoid

Sternothyroid

Sternocleidomastoid

Creek

Muscles of the Neck
Figure 13.10

Muscles of Inspiration

Muscles of Expiration

Sternocleidomastoid

Scalenes

External intercostals

Internal intercostals
(interchondral part)

Diaphragm

Creek

Internal intercostals
(excluding interchondral
part)

External abdominal oblique

Internal abdominal oblique

Transversus abdominis

Rectus abdominis

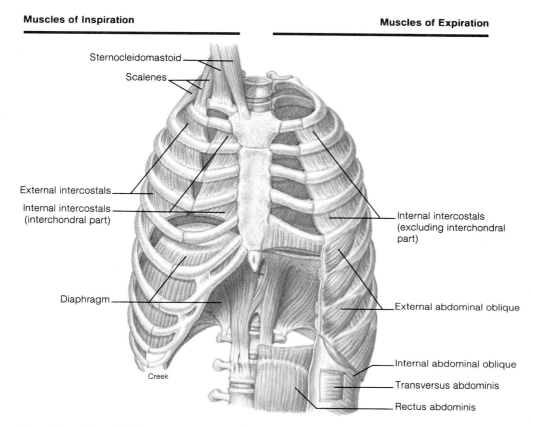

Muscles of Respiration
Figure 13.11

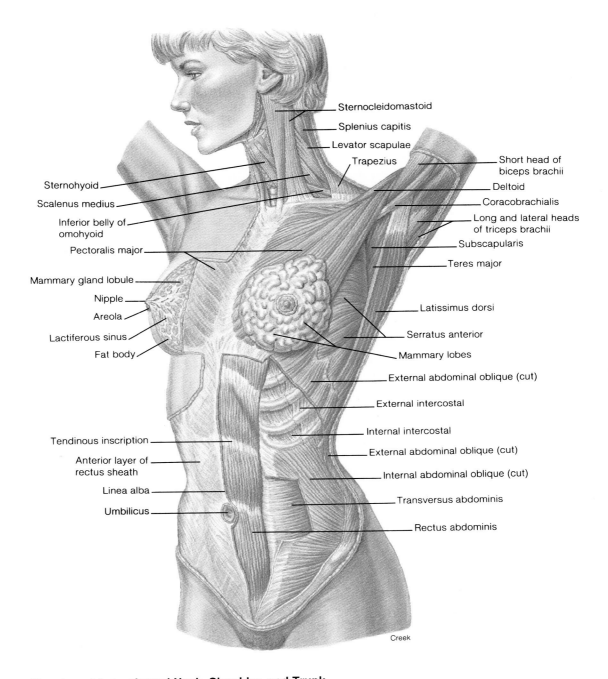

Sternocleidomastoid

Splenius capitis

Levator scapulae

Trapezius

Short head of biceps brachii

Deltoid

Coracobrachialis

Long and lateral heads of triceps brachii

Subscapularis

Teres major

Latissimus dorsi

Serratus anterior

Mammary lobes

External abdominal oblique (cut)

External intercostal

Internal intercostal

External abdominal oblique (cut)

Internal abdominal oblique (cut)

Transversus abdominis

Rectus abdominis

Sternohyoid

Scalenus medius

Inferior belly of omohyoid

Pectoralis major

Mammary gland lobule

Nipple

Areola

Lactiferous sinus

Fat body

Tendinous inscription

Anterior layer of rectus sheath

Linea alba

Umbilicus

Creek

Muscles of Anterolateral Neck, Shoulder, and Trunk
Figure 13.12

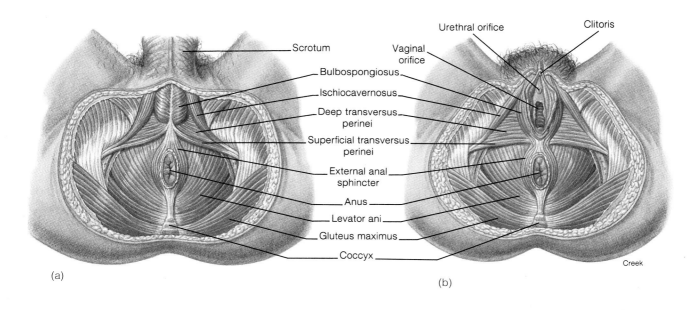

Scrotum

Urethral orifice
Clitoris
Vaginal orifice

Bulbospongiosus
Ischiocavernosus
Deep transversus perinei
Superficial transversus perinei
External anal sphincter
Anus
Levator ani
Gluteus maximus
Coccyx

Creek

(a)

(b)

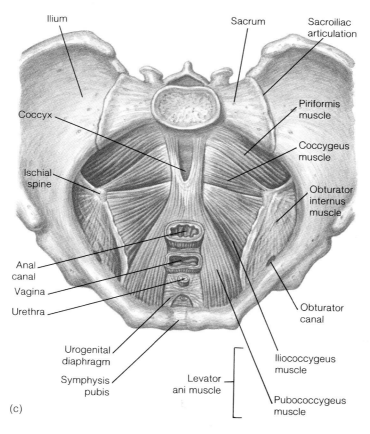

Ilium
Sacrum
Sacroiliac articulation

Coccyx

Piriformis muscle

Coccygeus muscle

Ischial spine

Obturator internus muscle

Anal canal
Vagina
Urethra

Urogenital diaphragm
Symphysis pubis

Obturator canal

Iliococcygeus muscle

Levator ani muscle

Pubococcygeus muscle

(c)

Muscles of Pelvic Outlet
Figure 13.13

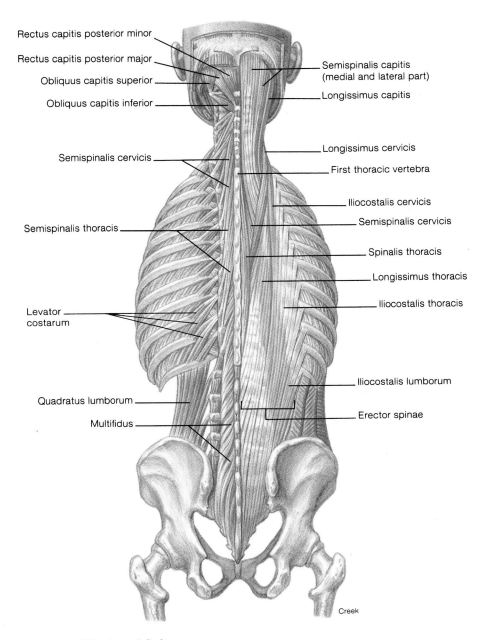

Rectus capitis posterior minor

Rectus capitis posterior major

Obliquus capitis superior

Obliquus capitis inferior

Semispinalis capitis
(medial and lateral part)

Longissimus capitis

Semispinalis cervicis

Longissimus cervicis

First thoracic vertebra

Iliocostalis cervicis

Semispinalis cervicis

Semispinalis thoracis

Spinalis thoracis

Longissimus thoracis

Iliocostalis thoracis

Levator
costarum

Iliocostalis lumborum

Quadratus lumborum

Erector spinae

Multifidus

Creek

Muscles of Vertebral Column
Figure 13.14

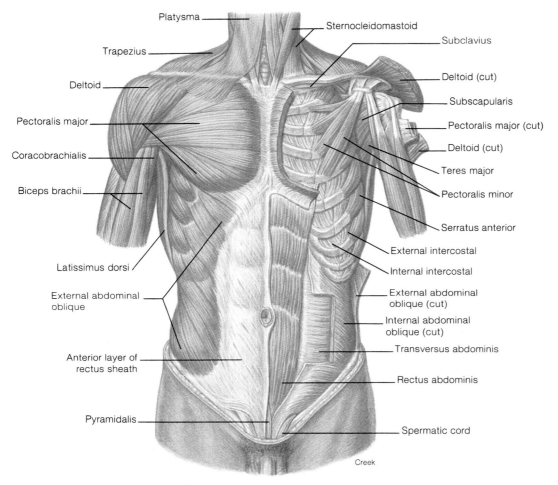

Platysma

Trapezius

Deltoid

Pectoralis major

Coracobrachialis

Biceps brachii

Latissimus dorsi

External abdominal oblique

Anterior layer of rectus sheath

Pyramidalis

Sternocleidomastoid

Subclavius

Deltoid (cut)

Subscapularis

Pectoralis major (cut)

Deltoid (cut)

Teres major

Pectoralis minor

Serratus anterior

External intercostal

Internal intercostal

External abdominal oblique (cut)

Internal abdominal oblique (cut)

Transversus abdominis

Rectus abdominis

Spermatic cord

Creek

Anterior Muscles of Trunk and Shoulder Regions
Figure 13.15

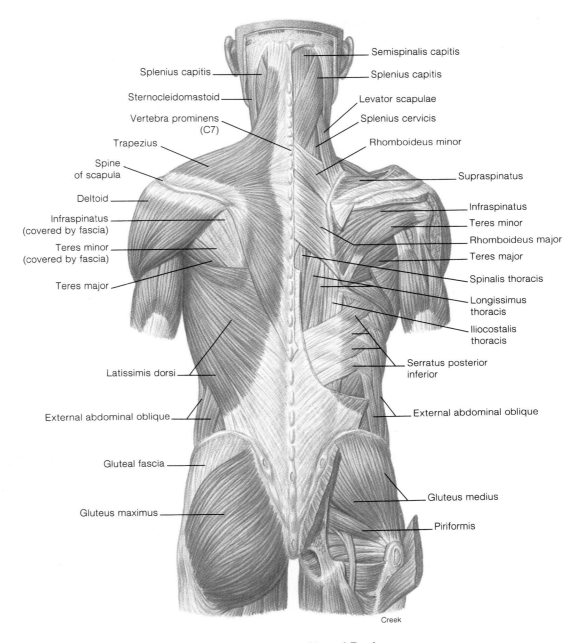

Semispinalis capitis

Splenius capitis

Splenius capitis

Sternocleidomastoid

Levator scapulae

Vertebra prominens
(C7)

Splenius cervicis

Trapezius

Rhomboideus minor

Spine
of scapula

Supraspinatus

Deltoid

Infraspinatus

Infraspinatus
(covered by fascia)

Teres minor

Rhomboideus major

Teres minor
(covered by fascia)

Teres major

Teres major

Spinalis thoracis

Longissimus
thoracis

Iliocostalis
thoracis

Latissimis dorsi

Serratus posterior
inferior

External abdominal oblique

External abdominal oblique

Gluteal fascia

Gluteus medius

Gluteus maximus

Piriformis

Creek

Posterior Muscles of Neck, Shoulder, Trunk, and Gluteal Regions
Figure 13.16

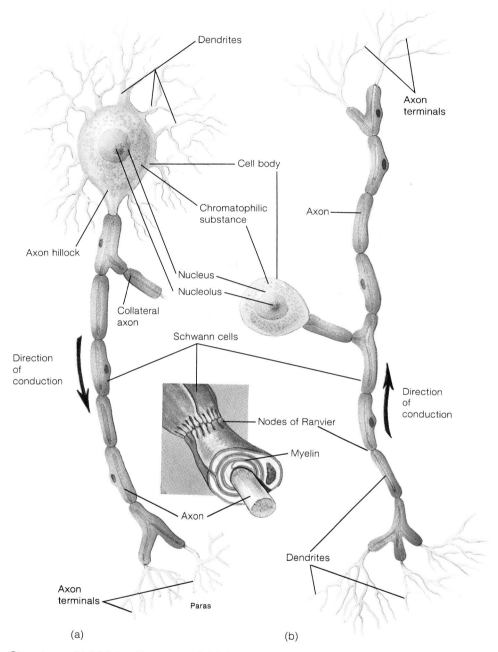

Dendrites

Axon
terminals

Cell body

Axon

Chromatophilic
substance

Axon hillock

Nucleus

Nucleolus

Collateral
axon

Schwann cells

Direction
of
conduction

Direction
of
conduction

Nodes of Ranvier

Myelin

Axon

Axon
terminals

Paras

Dendrites

(a)

(b)

Structure of (a) Motor Neuron and (b) Sensory Neuron
Figure 14.1

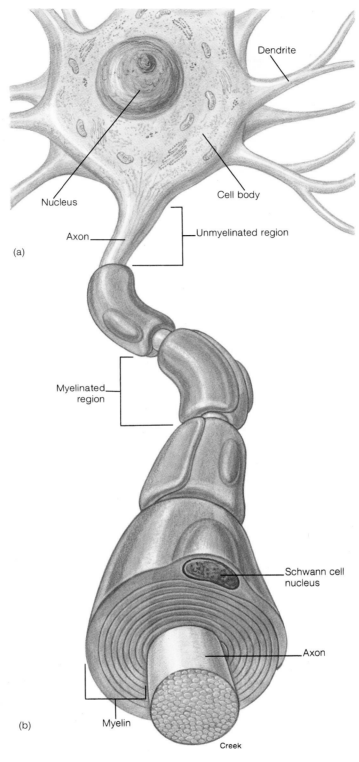

(a)

Dendrite

Nucleus

Cell body

Axon

Unmyelinated region

Myelinated region

Schwann cell nucleus

Axon

(b)

Myelin

Creek

A Myelinated Neuron
Figure 14.5

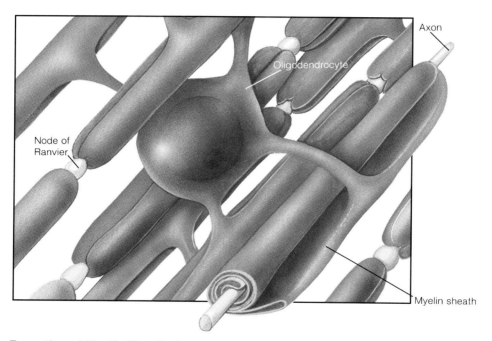

Formation of Myelin Sheaths in the Central Nervous System
Figure 14.8

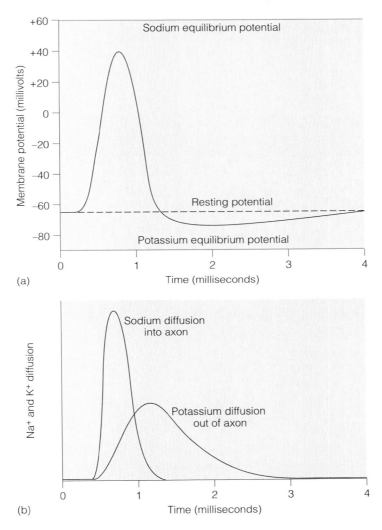

An Action Potential
Figure 14.12

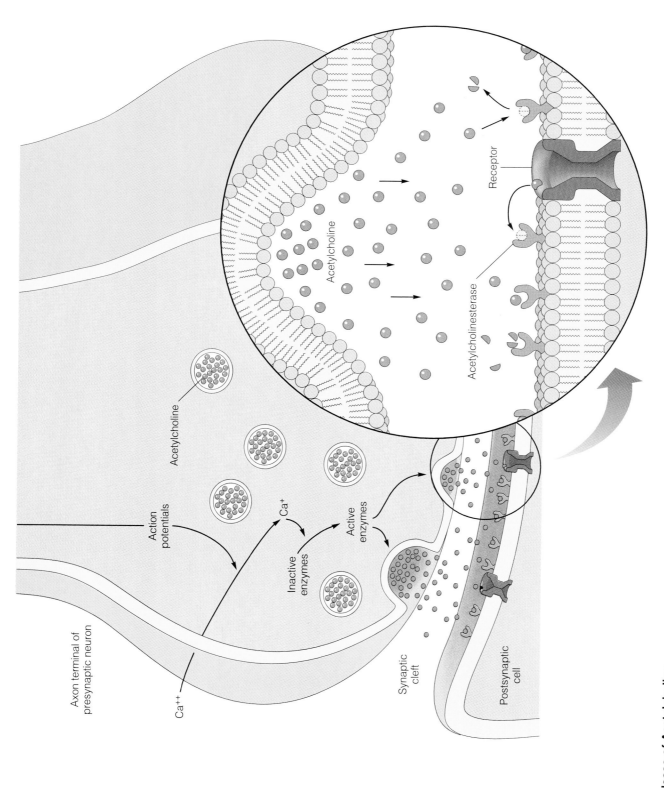

Axon terminal of
presynaptic neuron

Ca⁺⁺

Action
potentials

Acetylcholine

Ca⁺

Inactive
enzymes

Active
enzymes

Acetylcholine

Acetylcholinesterase

Receptor

Synaptic
cleft

Postsynaptic
cell

The Release of Acetylcholine
Figure 14.21

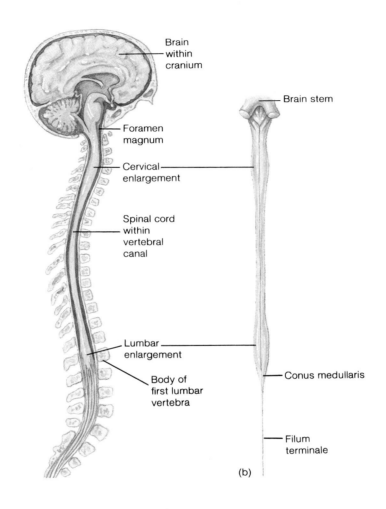

Brain within cranium

Brain stem

Foramen magnum

Cervical enlargement

Spinal cord within vertebral canal

Lumbar enlargement

Body of first lumbar vertebra

Conus medullaris

Filum terminale

(b)

(a)

Central Nervous System
Figure 15.1

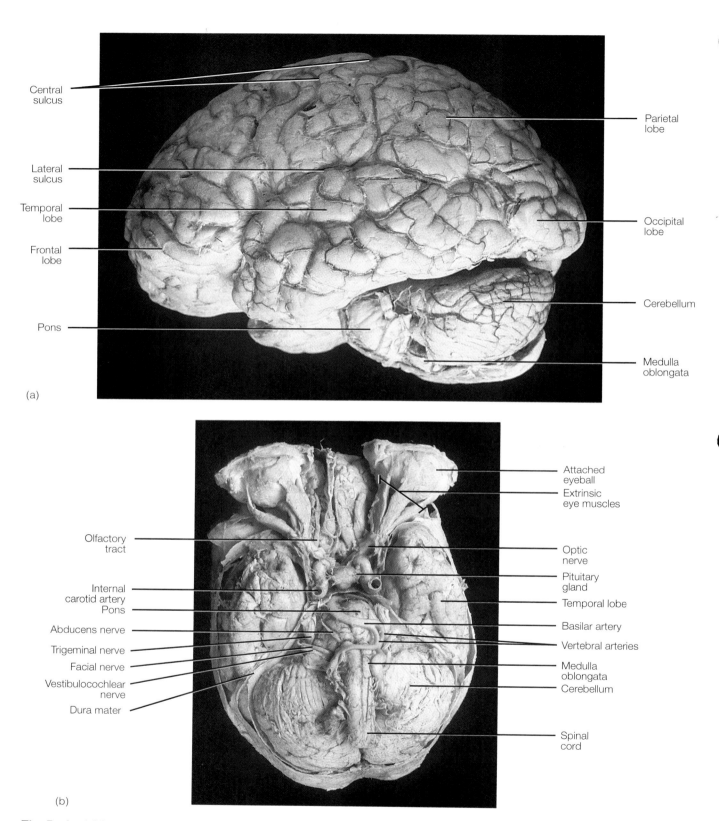

Central sulcus

Lateral sulcus

Temporal lobe

Frontal lobe

Pons

Parietal lobe

Occipital lobe

Cerebellum

Medulla oblongata

(a)

Olfactory tract

Internal carotid artery
Pons

Abducens nerve

Trigeminal nerve

Facial nerve

Vestibulocochlear nerve

Dura mater

Attached eyeball

Extrinsic eye muscles

Optic nerve

Pituitary gland

Temporal lobe

Basilar artery

Vertebral arteries

Medulla oblongata
Cerebellum

Spinal cord

(b)

The Brain. (a) Lateral View, (b) Inferior View, and (c) Sagittal View
Figure 15.3a,b,and c

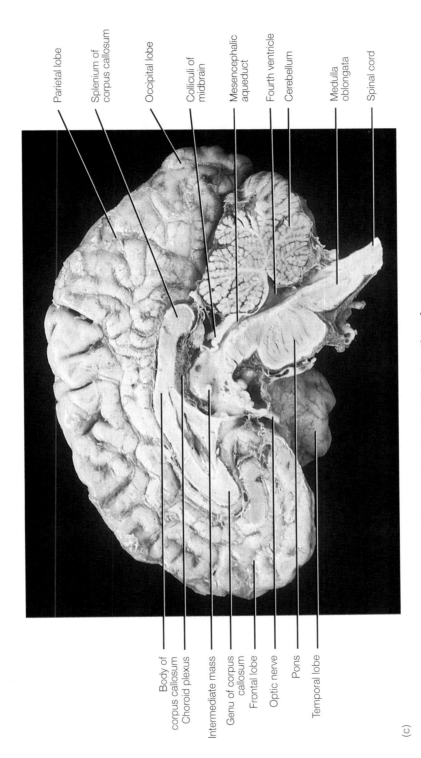

Parietal lobe

Splenium of
corpus callosum

Occipital lobe

Colliculi of
midbrain

Mesencephalic
aqueduct

Fourth ventricle

Cerebellum

Medulla
oblongata

Spinal cord

Body of
corpus callosum

Choroid plexus

Intermediate mass

Genu of corpus
callosum

Frontal lobe

Optic nerve

Pons

Temporal lobe

(c)

The Brain. (a) Lateral View, (b) Inferior View, and (c) Sagittal View (*continued*)
Figure 15.3a,b,and c

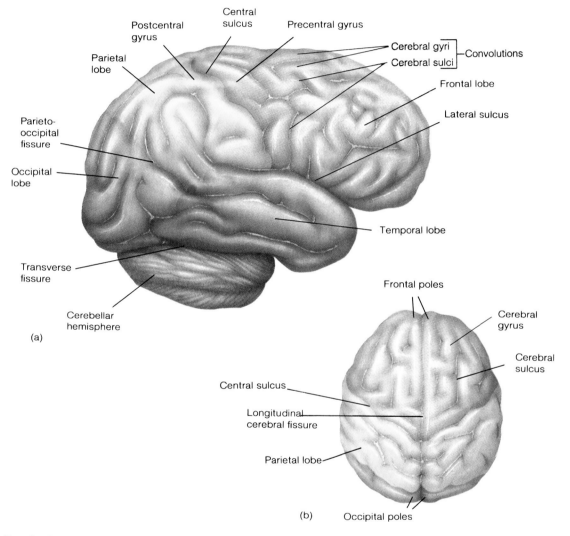

Central
sulcus

Postcentral
gyrus

Precentral gyrus

Parietal
lobe

Cerebral gyri
Cerebral sulci

Convolutions

Frontal lobe

Parieto-
occipital
fissure

Lateral sulcus

Occipital
lobe

Transverse
fissure

Temporal lobe

Cerebellar
hemisphere

(a)

Frontal poles

Cerebral
gyrus

Cerebral
sulcus

Central sulcus

Longitudinal
cerebral fissure

Parietal lobe

(b)   Occipital poles

Cerebral Lobes
Figure 15.4

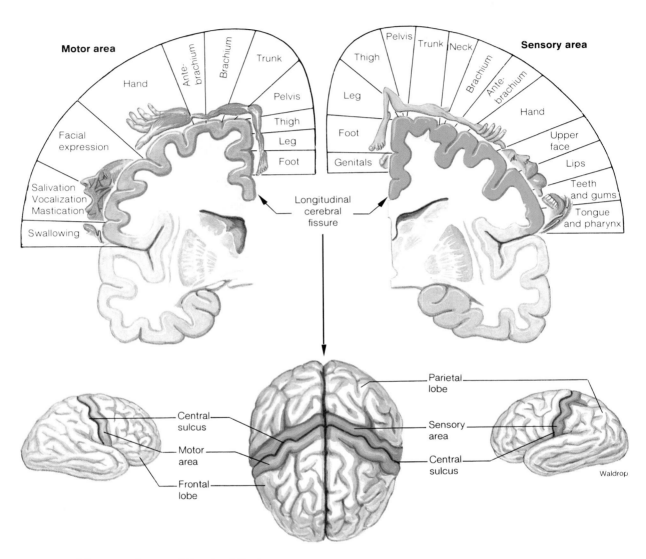

Motor and Sensory Areas of Cerebral Cortex
Figure 15.7

63

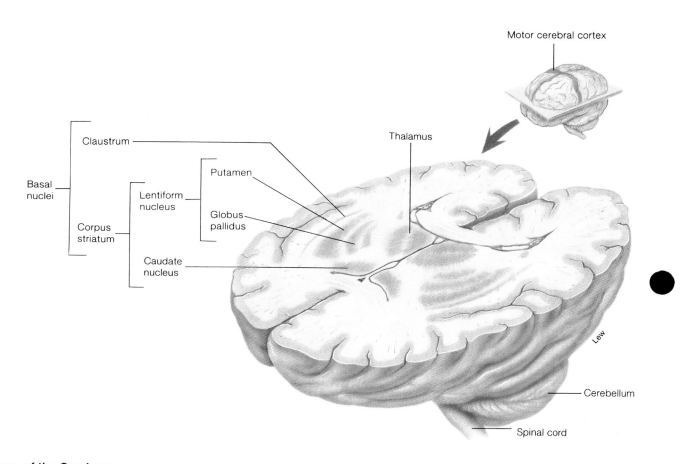

Motor cerebral cortex

Thalamus

Claustrum

Basal nuclei

Putamen

Lentiform nucleus

Corpus striatum

Globus pallidus

Caudate nucleus

Lew

Cerebellum

Spinal cord

Structures of the Cerebrum
Figure 15.11

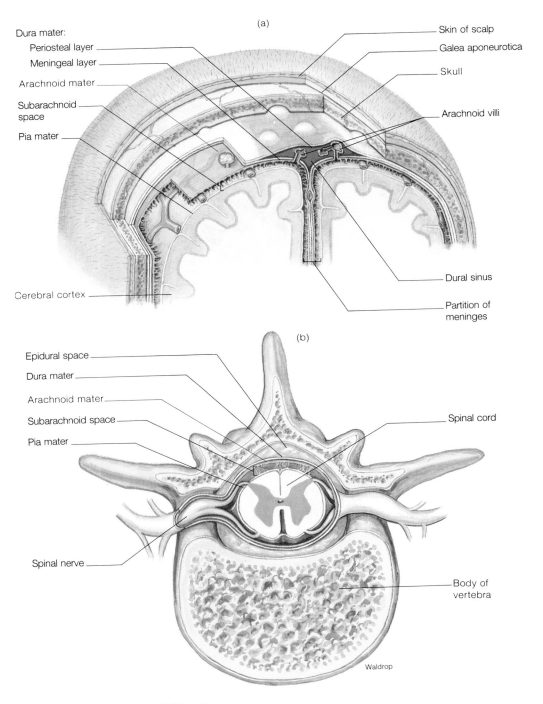

(a)

Dura mater:
Periosteal layer
Meningeal layer
Arachnoid mater
Subarachnoid space
Pia mater

Skin of scalp
Galea aponeurotica
Skull
Arachnoid villi

Cerebral cortex

Dural sinus

Partition of meninges

(b)

Epidural space
Dura mater
Arachnoid mater
Subarachnoid space
Pia mater

Spinal cord

Spinal nerve

Body of vertebra

Waldrop

Meninges and Associated Structures
Figure 15.19

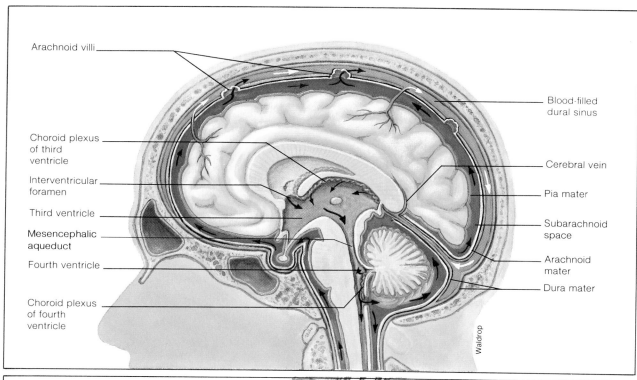

Arachnoid villi

Choroid plexus of third ventricle

Interventricular foramen

Third ventricle

Mesencephalic aqueduct

Fourth ventricle

Choroid plexus of fourth ventricle

Blood-filled dural sinus

Cerebral vein

Pia mater

Subarachnoid space

Arachnoid mater

Dura mater

Waldrop

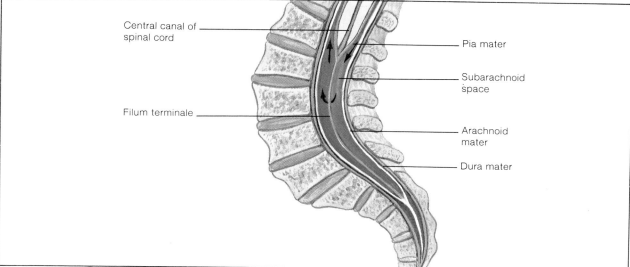

Central canal of spinal cord

Filum terminale

Pia mater

Subarachnoid space

Arachnoid mater

Dura mater

Meninges and Cerebrospinal Fluid
Figure 15.22

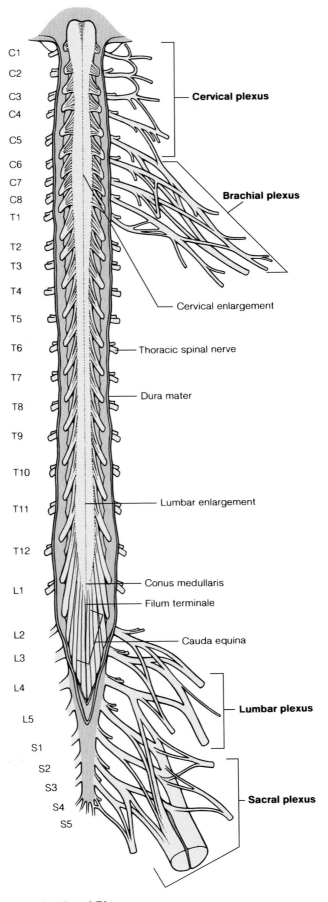

C1
C2
C3
C4
C5
C6
C7
C8
T1
T2
T3
T4
T5
T6
T7
T8
T9
T10
T11
T12
L1
L2
L3
L4
L5
S1
S2
S3
S4
S5

Cervical plexus

Brachial plexus

Cervical enlargement

Thoracic spinal nerve

Dura mater

Lumbar enlargement

Conus medullaris

Filum terminale

Cauda equina

Lumbar plexus

Sacral plexus

Spinal Cord and Plexuses
Figure 15.23

67

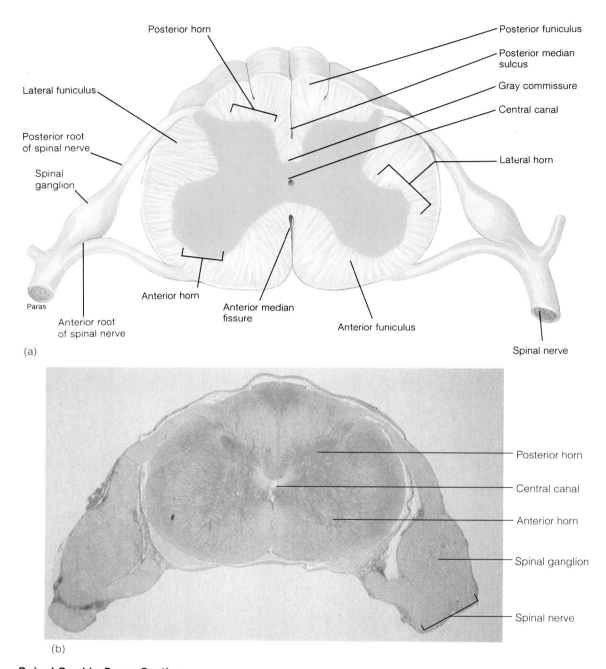

Posterior horn

Posterior funiculus

Posterior median sulcus

Lateral funiculus

Gray commissure

Central canal

Posterior root of spinal nerve

Spinal ganglion

Lateral horn

Paras

Anterior horn

Anterior median fissure

Anterior funiculus

Anterior root of spinal nerve

Spinal nerve

(a)

(b)

Posterior horn

Central canal

Anterior horn

Spinal ganglion

Spinal nerve

Spinal Cord in Cross Section
Figure 15.24a,b

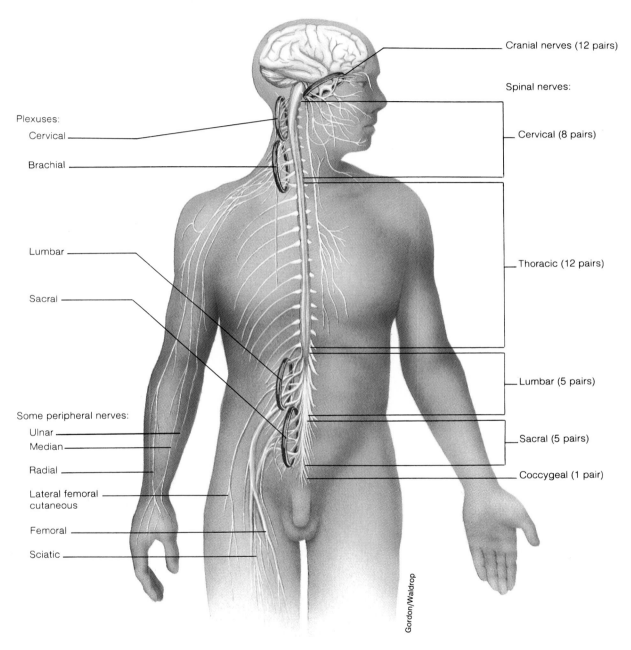

Cranial nerves (12 pairs)

Spinal nerves:

Cervical (8 pairs)

Thoracic (12 pairs)

Lumbar (5 pairs)

Sacral (5 pairs)

Coccygeal (1 pair)

Plexuses:
Cervical
Brachial
Lumbar
Sacral

Some peripheral nerves:
Ulnar
Median
Radial
Lateral femoral cutaneous
Femoral
Sciatic

Gordon/Waldrop

The Peripheral Nervous System
Figure 16.1

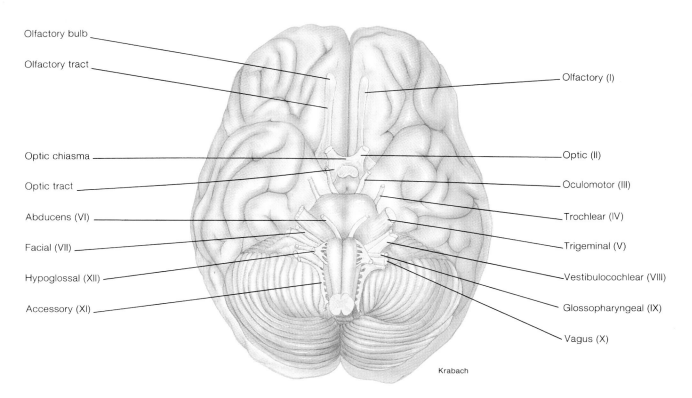

Olfactory bulb
Olfactory tract
Optic chiasma
Optic tract
Abducens (VI)
Facial (VII)
Hypoglossal (XII)
Accessory (XI)

Olfactory (I)
Optic (II)
Oculomotor (III)
Trochlear (IV)
Trigeminal (V)
Vestibulocochlear (VIII)
Glossopharyngeal (IX)
Vagus (X)

Krabach

Cranial Nerves
Figure 16.3

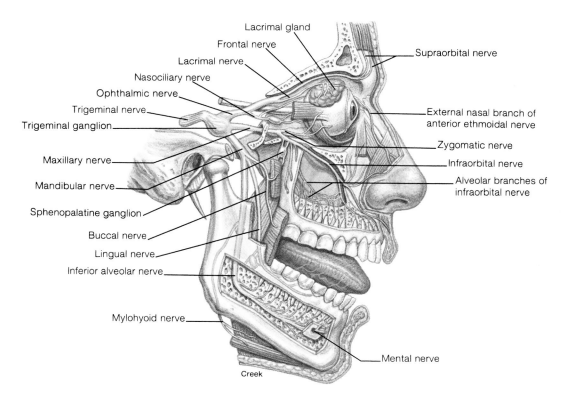

Lacrimal gland
Frontal nerve
Lacrimal nerve
Nasociliary nerve
Ophthalmic nerve
Trigeminal nerve
Trigeminal ganglion
Maxillary nerve
Mandibular nerve
Sphenopalatine ganglion
Buccal nerve
Lingual nerve
Inferior alveolar nerve
Mylohyoid nerve

Supraorbital nerve
External nasal branch of anterior ethmoidal nerve
Zygomatic nerve
Infraorbital nerve
Alveolar branches of infraorbital nerve
Mental nerve

Creek

Trigeminal Nerve
Figure 16.7

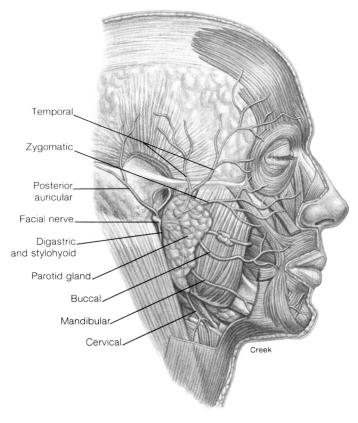

Temporal

Zygomatic

Posterior auricular

Facial nerve

Digastric and stylohyoid

Parotid gland

Buccal

Mandibular

Cervical

Creek

Facial Nerve
Figure 16.8

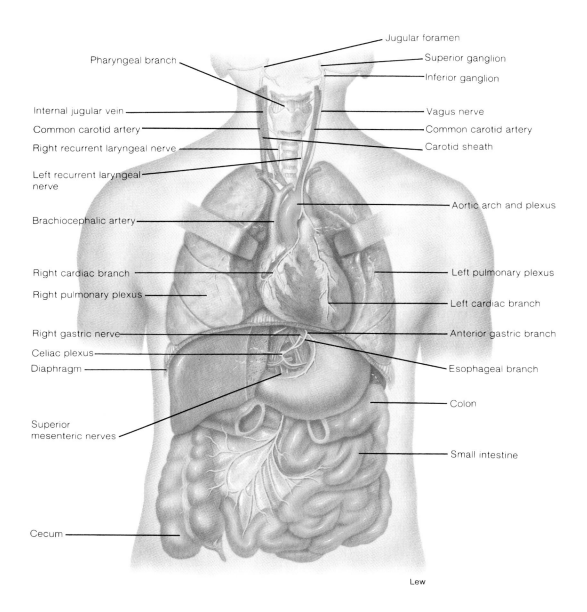

Pharyngeal branch

Internal jugular vein
Common carotid artery
Right recurrent laryngeal nerve
Left recurrent laryngeal nerve

Brachiocephalic artery

Right cardiac branch
Right pulmonary plexus

Right gastric nerve
Celiac plexus
Diaphragm

Superior mesenteric nerves

Cecum

Jugular foramen
Superior ganglion
Inferior ganglion

Vagus nerve
Common carotid artery
Carotid sheath

Aortic arch and plexus

Left pulmonary plexus

Left cardiac branch

Anterior gastric branch

Esophageal branch

Colon

Small intestine

Lew

Vagus Nerve
Figure 16.11

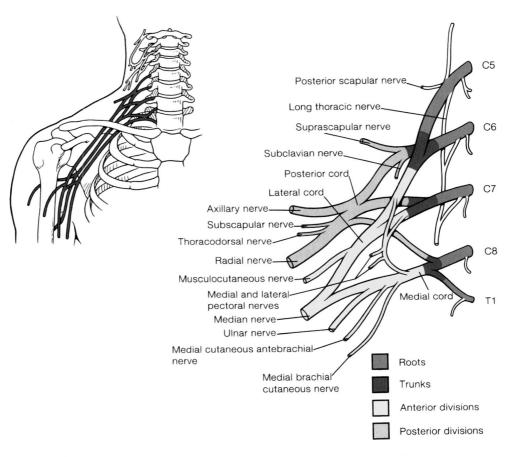

Posterior scapular nerve
Long thoracic nerve
Suprascapular nerve
Subclavian nerve
Posterior cord
Lateral cord
Axillary nerve
Subscapular nerve
Thoracodorsal nerve
Radial nerve
Musculocutaneous nerve
Medial and lateral pectoral nerves
Median nerve
Ulnar nerve
Medial cutaneous antebrachial nerve
Medial brachial cutaneous nerve

C5
C6
C7
C8
T1

Medial cord

Roots
Trunks
Anterior divisions
Posterior divisions

Brachial Plexus
Figure 16.15

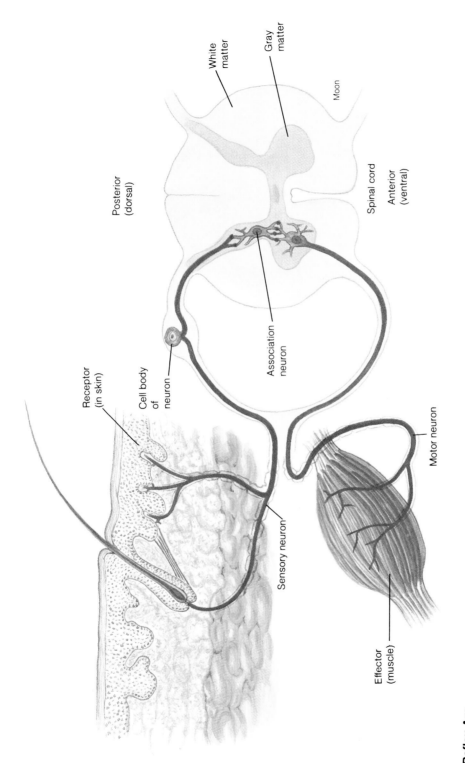

White matter

Gray matter

Moon

Posterior
(dorsal)

Spinal cord

Anterior
(ventral)

Receptor
(in skin)

Cell body
of
neuron

Association
neuron

Sensory neuron

Motor neuron

Effector
(muscle)

Reflex Arc
Figure 16.28

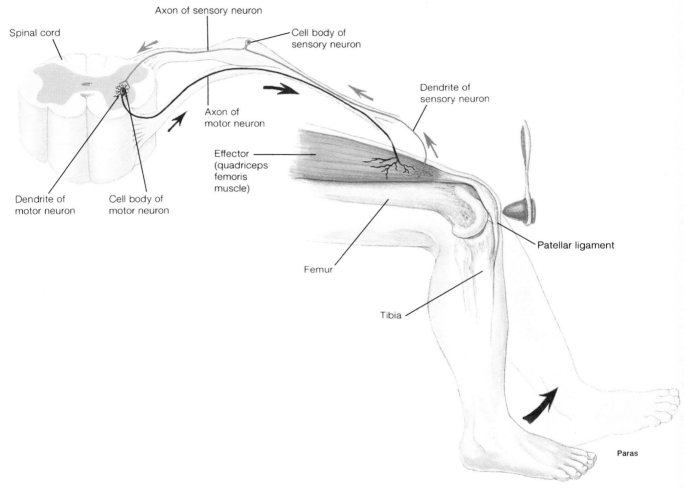

Spinal cord

Axon of sensory neuron

Cell body of
sensory neuron

Dendrite of
sensory neuron

Axon of
motor neuron

Effector
(quadriceps
femoris
muscle)

Dendrite of
motor neuron

Cell body of
motor neuron

Femur

Patellar ligament

Tibia

Paras

Knee-Jerk Reflex
Figure 16.29

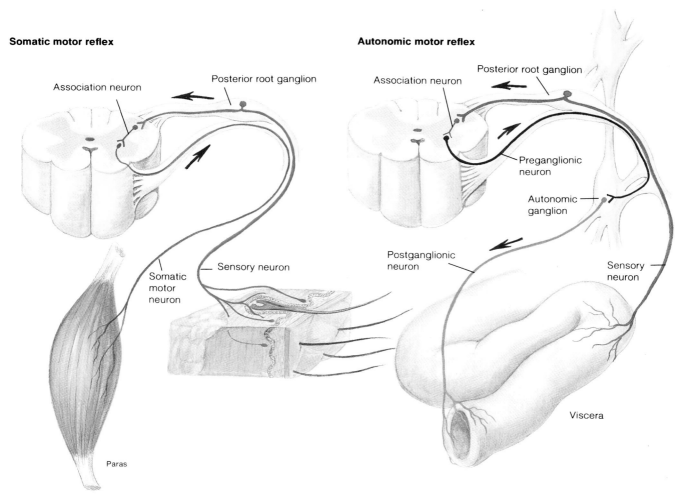

Somatic motor reflex

Association neuron

Posterior root ganglion

Somatic motor neuron

Sensory neuron

Paras

Autonomic motor reflex

Association neuron

Posterior root ganglion

Preganglionic neuron

Autonomic ganglion

Postganglionic neuron

Sensory neuron

Viscera

Comparison of a Somatic Motor Reflex and an Autonomic Motor Reflex
Figure 17.1

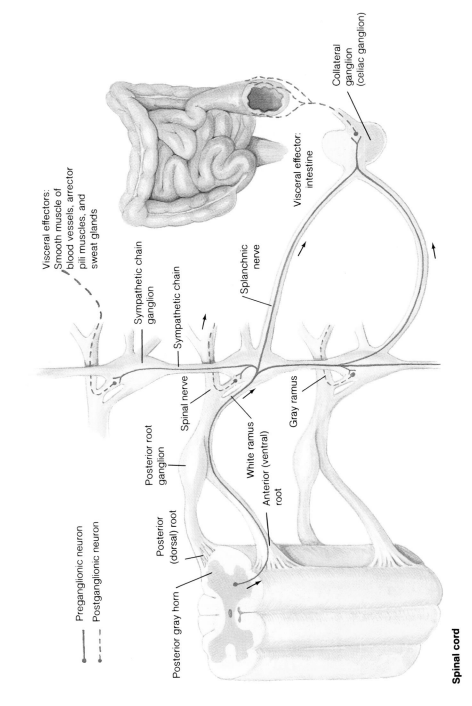

Visceral effectors:
Smooth muscle of
blood vessels, arrector
pili muscles, and
sweat glands

Sympathetic chain
ganglion

Sympathetic chain

Splanchnic
nerve

Visceral effector:
intestine

Collateral
ganglion
(celiac ganglion)

Spinal nerve

White ramus

Anterior (ventral)
root

Gray ramus

Posterior root
ganglion

Posterior
(dorsal) root

Posterior gray horn

Preganglionic neuron
Postganglionic neuron

Spinal cord

Sympathetic Chain Ganglia
Figure 17.3

77

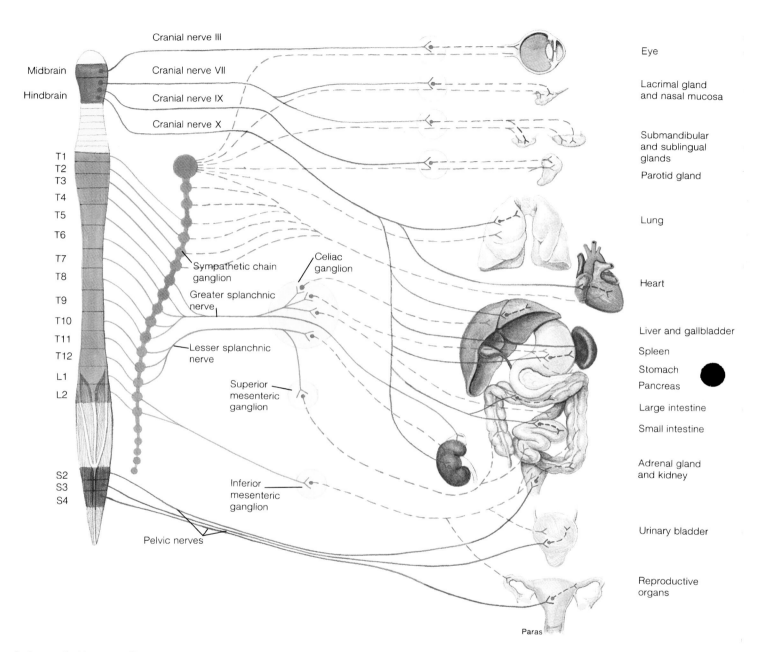

Cranial nerve III

Midbrain

Cranial nerve VII

Hindbrain

Cranial nerve IX

Cranial nerve X

T1
T2
T3
T4
T5
T6
T7
T8
T9
T10
T11
T12
L1
L2

Sympathetic chain ganglion

Celiac ganglion

Greater splanchnic nerve

Lesser splanchnic nerve

Superior mesenteric ganglion

S2
S3
S4

Inferior mesenteric ganglion

Pelvic nerves

Eye

Lacrimal gland and nasal mucosa

Submandibular and sublingual glands

Parotid gland

Lung

Heart

Liver and gallbladder

Spleen

Stomach

Pancreas

Large intestine

Small intestine

Adrenal gland and kidney

Urinary bladder

Reproductive organs

Paras

Autonomic Nervous System
Figure 17.7

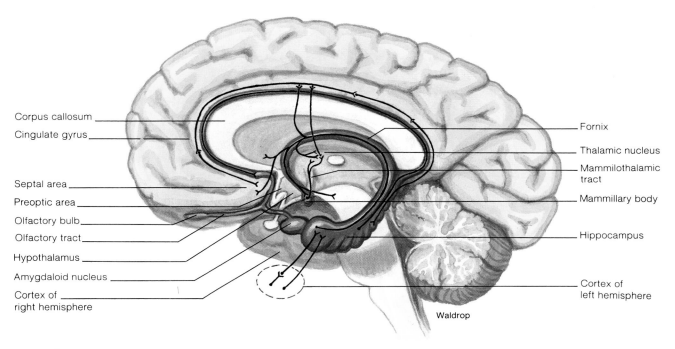

Corpus callosum

Cingulate gyrus

Septal area

Preoptic area

Olfactory bulb

Olfactory tract

Hypothalamus

Amygdaloid nucleus

Cortex of
right hemisphere

Fornix

Thalamic nucleus

Mammilothalamic
tract

Mammillary body

Hippocampus

Cortex of
left hemisphere

Waldrop

Limbic System
Figure 17.10

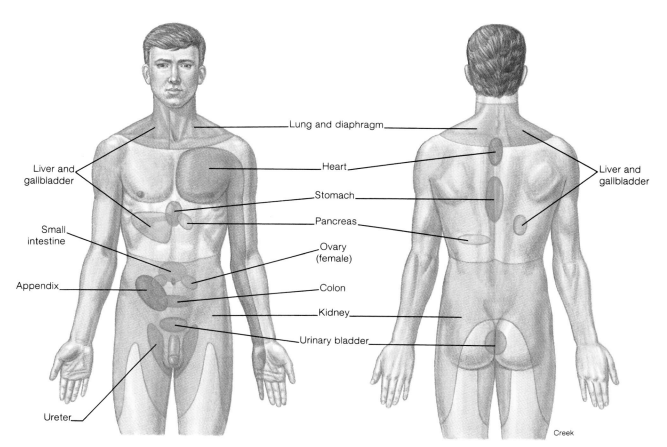

Sites of Referred Pain
Figure 18.3

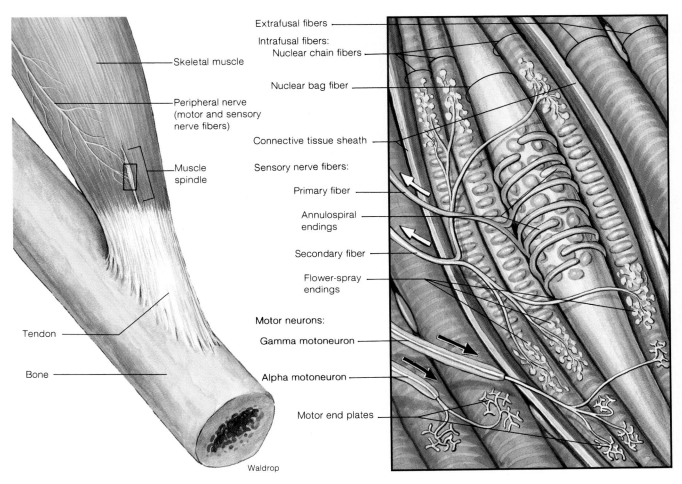

Extrafusal fibers

Intrafusal fibers:
Nuclear chain fibers

Nuclear bag fiber

Connective tissue sheath

Sensory nerve fibers:

Primary fiber

Annulospiral endings

Secondary fiber

Flower-spray endings

Motor neurons:

Gamma motoneuron

Alpha motoneuron

Motor end plates

Skeletal muscle

Peripheral nerve (motor and sensory nerve fibers)

Muscle spindle

Tendon

Bone

Waldrop

Structure of Muscle Spindles
Figure 18.5

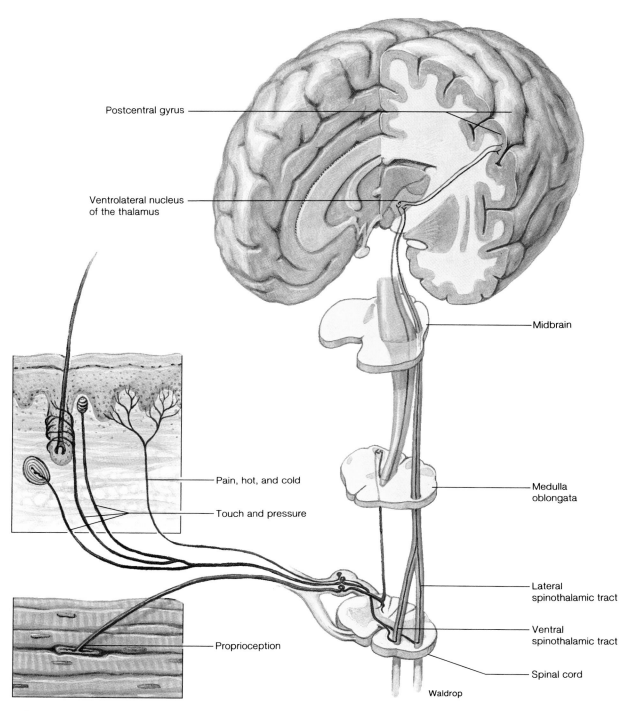

Postcentral gyrus

Ventrolateral nucleus
of the thalamus

Pain, hot, and cold

Touch and pressure

Proprioception

Midbrain

Medulla
oblongata

Lateral
spinothalamic tract

Ventral
spinothalamic tract

Spinal cord

Waldrop

Sensory Pathways to Brain
Figure 18.8

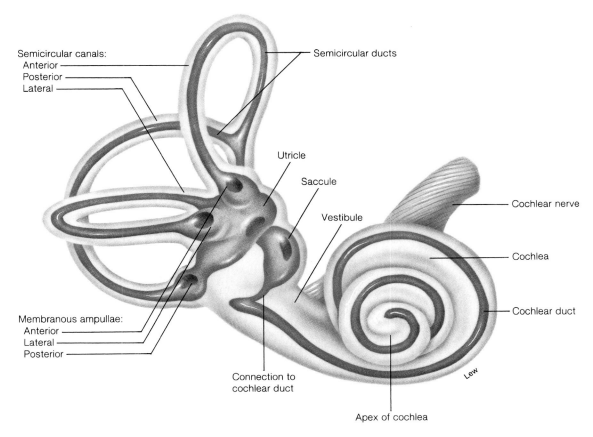

Semicircular canals:
Anterior
Posterior
Lateral

Semicircular ducts

Utricle

Saccule

Vestibule

Cochlear nerve

Cochlea

Cochlear duct

Membranous ampullae:
Anterior
Lateral
Posterior

Connection to
cochlear duct

Lew

Apex of cochlea

Labyrinths of Inner Ear
Figure 18.13

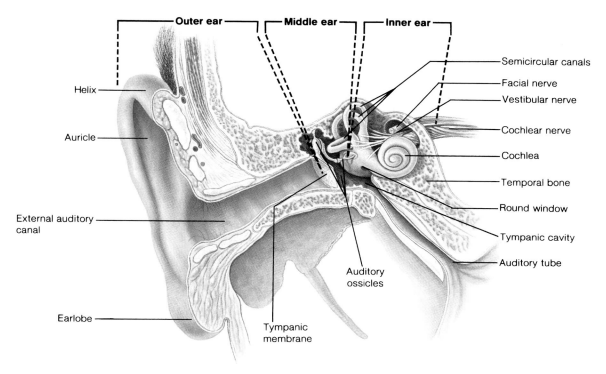

Outer ear   Middle ear   Inner ear

Helix

Auricle

External auditory
canal

Earlobe

Semicircular canals

Facial nerve

Vestibular nerve

Cochlear nerve

Cochlea

Temporal bone

Round window

Tympanic cavity

Auditory tube

Auditory
ossicles

Tympanic
membrane

Structure of the Ear
Figure 18.19

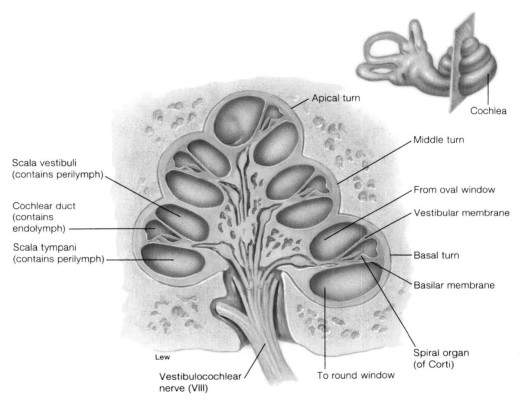

Apical turn

Middle turn

Cochlea

Scala vestibuli
(contains perilymph)

From oval window

Vestibular membrane

Cochlear duct
(contains
endolymph)

Basal turn

Scala tympani
(contains perilymph)

Basilar membrane

Lew

Spiral organ
(of Corti)

Vestibulocochlear
nerve (VIII)

To round window

Structure of the Cochlea
Figure 18.21

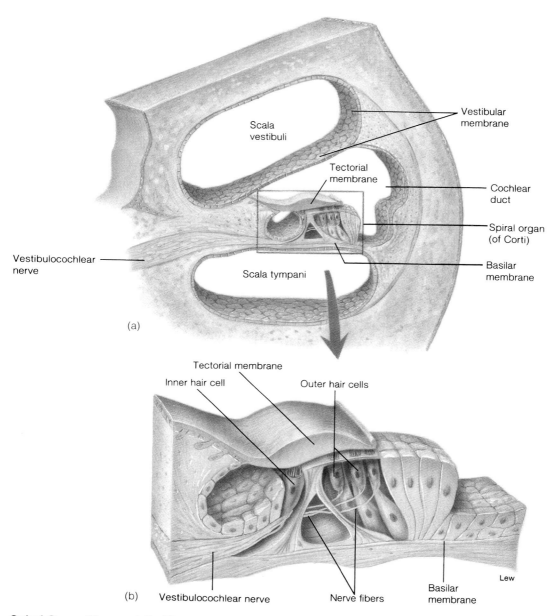

Scala
vestibuli

Vestibular
membrane

Tectorial
membrane

Cochlear
duct

Spiral organ
(of Corti)

Basilar
membrane

Vestibulocochlear
nerve

Scala tympani

(a)

Tectorial membrane

Inner hair cell

Outer hair cells

Lew

(b)   Vestibulocochlear nerve   Nerve fibers   Basilar
membrane

Spiral Organ (Organ of Corti)
Figure 18.23

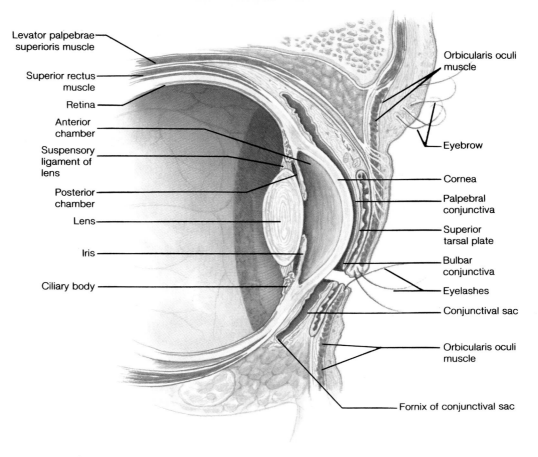

Accessory Structures of Eyeball
Figure 18.28

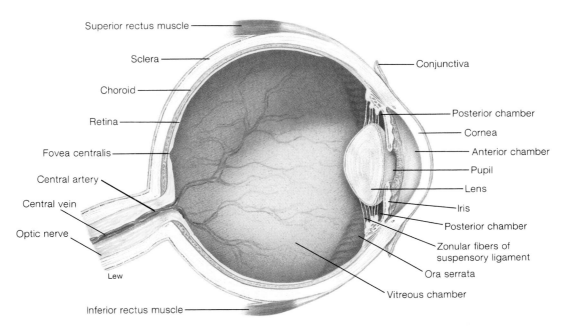

Internal Anatomy of Eye
Figure 18.29

87

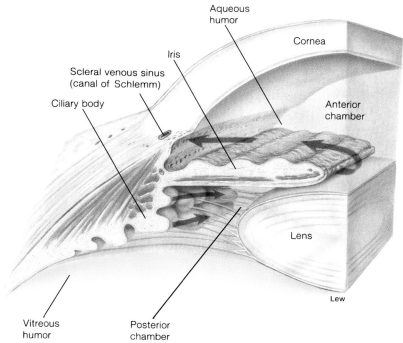

Flow of Aqueous Humor
Figure 18.31

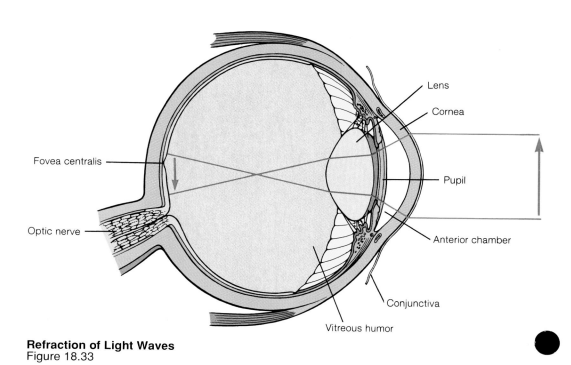

Refraction of Light Waves
Figure 18.33

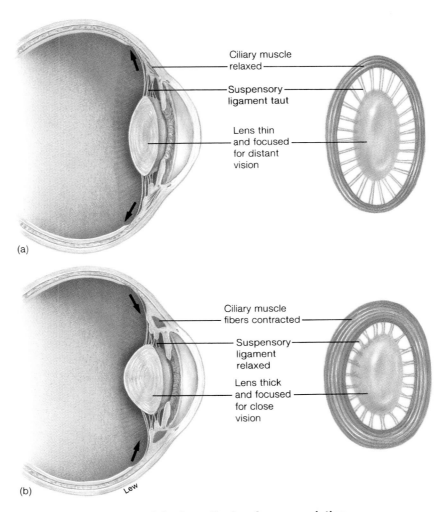

Changes in the Shape of the Lens During Accommodation
Figure 18.36

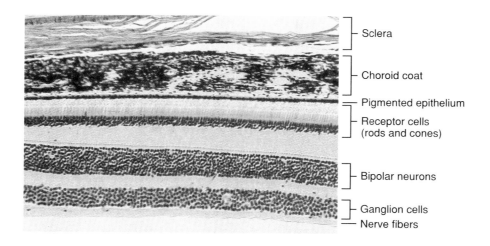

Sclera

Choroid coat

Pigmented epithelium

Receptor cells
(rods and cones)

Bipolar neurons

Ganglion cells

Nerve fibers

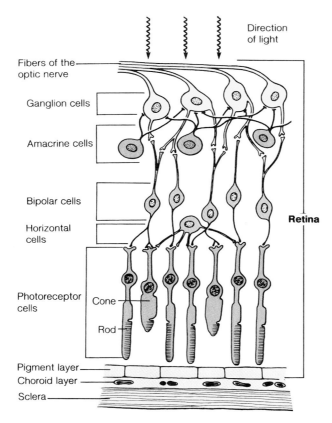

Direction
of light

Fibers of the
optic nerve

Ganglion cells

Amacrine cells

Bipolar cells

Horizontal
cells

Retina

Photoreceptor
cells

Cone

Rod

Pigment layer

Choroid layer

Sclera

Layers of Retina
Figures 18.37 and 18.38

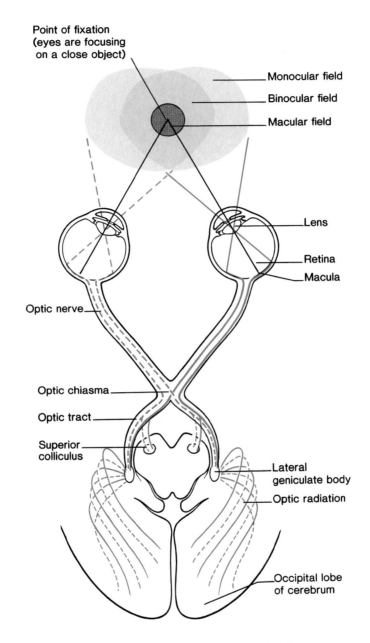

Point of fixation
(eyes are focusing
on a close object)

Monocular field

Binocular field

Macular field

Lens

Retina

Macula

Optic nerve

Optic chiasma

Optic tract

Superior colliculus

Lateral geniculate body

Optic radiation

Occipital lobe of cerebrum

Visual Fields and the Neural Pathways for Vision
Figure 18.44

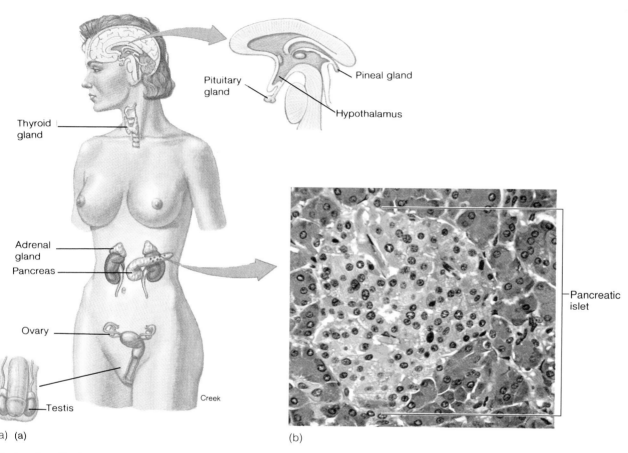

Thyroid
gland

Pituitary
gland

Pineal gland

Hypothalamus

Adrenal
gland

Pancreas

Ovary

Creek

Testis

Pancreatic
islet

(a) (a)

(b)

Endocrine System
Figure 19.1

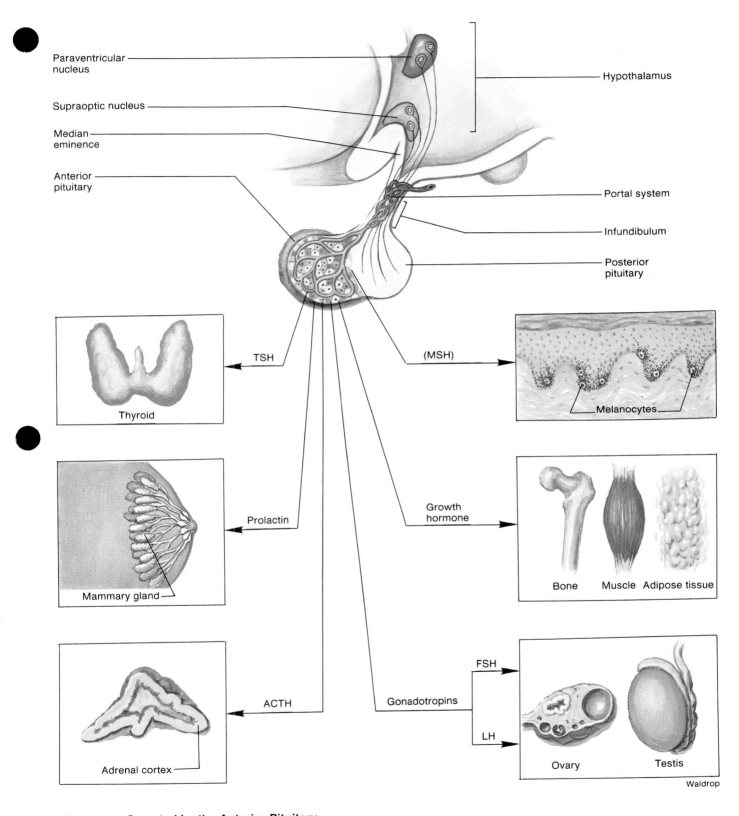

Paraventricular nucleus

Supraoptic nucleus

Median eminence

Anterior pituitary

Hypothalamus

Portal system

Infundibulum

Posterior pituitary

TSH

Thyroid

(MSH)

Melanocytes

Prolactin

Mammary gland

Growth hormone

Bone   Muscle   Adipose tissue

ACTH

Adrenal cortex

Gonadotropins

FSH

LH

Ovary   Testis

Waldrop

Hormones Secreted by the Anterior Pituitary
Figure 19.6

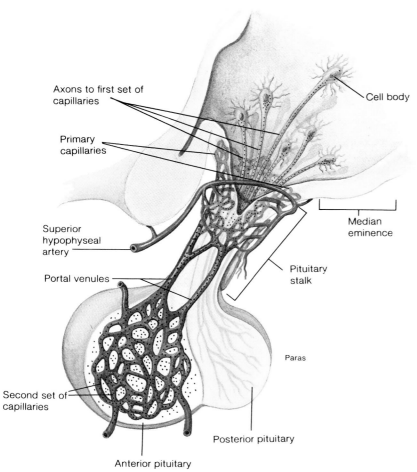

Axons to first set of
capillaries

Cell body

Primary
capillaries

Median
eminence

Superior
hypophyseal
artery

Pituitary
stalk

Portal venules

Paras

Second set of
capillaries

Posterior pituitary

Anterior pituitary

Hypothalmo-hypophyseal Portal System
Figure 19.7

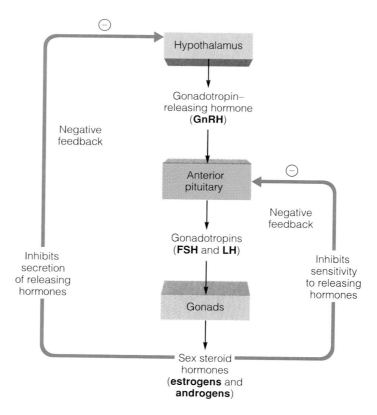

Hypothalamus

⊖ Negative feedback

Gonadotropin–
releasing hormone
(**GnRH**)

Inhibits
secretion
of releasing
hormones

Anterior
pituitary

⊖ Negative feedback

Gonadotropins
(**FSH** and **LH**)

Inhibits
sensitivity
to releasing
hormones

Gonads

Sex steroid
hormones
(**estrogens** and
androgens)

Negative Feedback Control of Gonadotropin Secretion
Figure 19.9

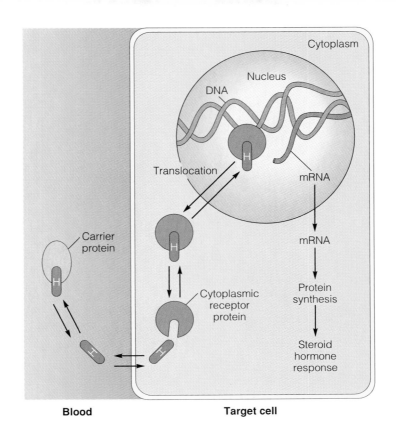

The Action of a Steroid Hormone
Figure 19.21

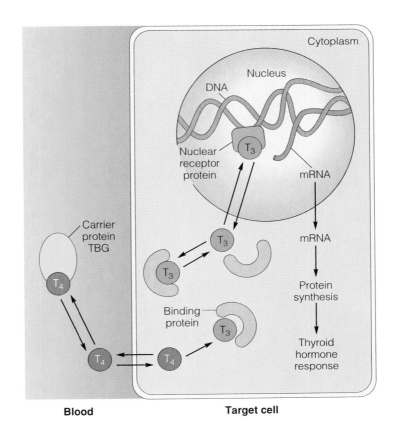

Cyclic AMP as a Second Messenger
Figure 19.22

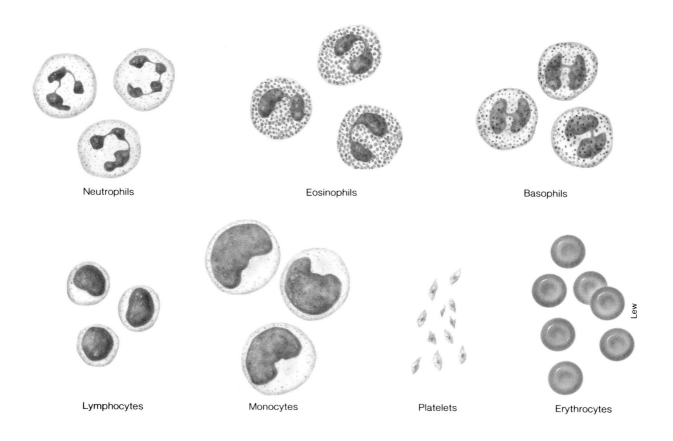

Neutrophils

Eosinophils

Basophils

Lymphocytes

Monocytes

Platelets

Erythrocytes

Formed Elements of the Blood
Figure 20.3

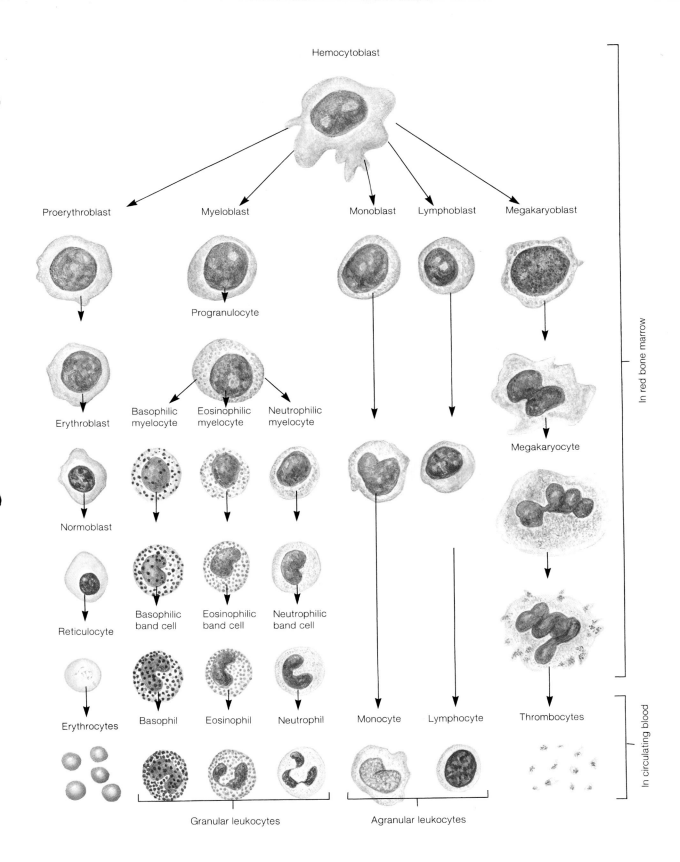

Hemocytoblast

Proerythroblast Myeloblast Monoblast Lymphoblast Megakaryoblast

Progranulocyte

Erythroblast Basophilic Eosinophilic Neutrophilic
myelocyte myelocyte myelocyte

Megakaryocyte

Normoblast

Reticulocyte Basophilic Eosinophilic Neutrophilic
band cell band cell band cell

Erythrocytes Basophil Eosinophil Neutrophil Monocyte Lymphocyte Thrombocytes

Granular leukocytes Agranular leukocytes

In red bone marrow

In circulating blood

Process of Hemopoiesis
Figure 20.4

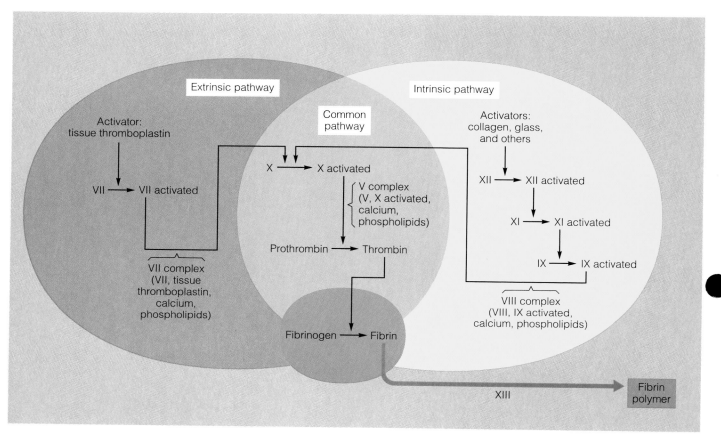

Extrinsic and Intrinsic Clotting Pathways
Figure 20.8

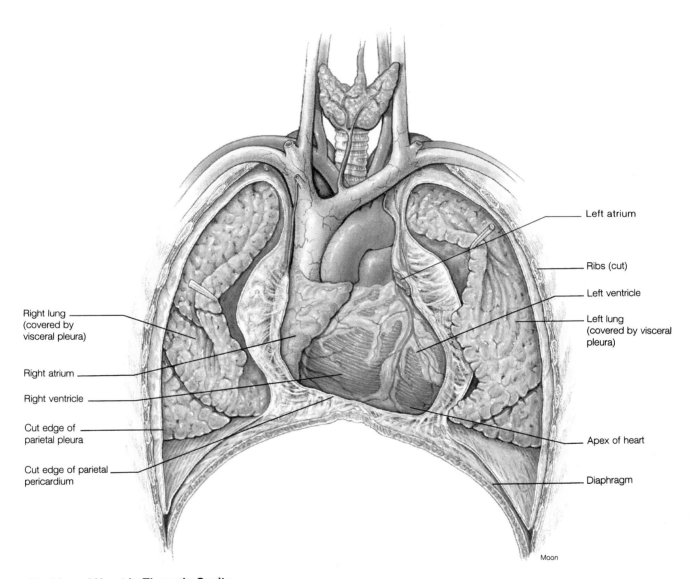

Right lung
(covered by
visceral pleura)

Right atrium

Right ventricle

Cut edge of
parietal pleura

Cut edge of parietal
pericardium

Left atrium

Ribs (cut)

Left ventricle

Left lung
(covered by visceral
pleura)

Apex of heart

Diaphragm

Moon

Position of Heart in Thoracic Cavity
Figure 21.1

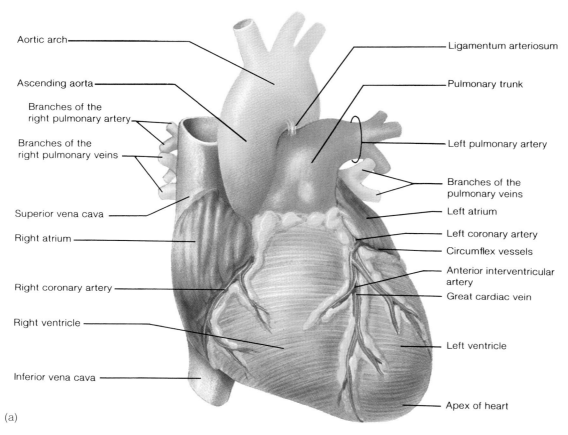

Aortic arch

Ascending aorta

Branches of the
right pulmonary artery

Branches of the
right pulmonary veins

Superior vena cava

Right atrium

Right coronary artery

Right ventricle

Inferior vena cava

Ligamentum arteriosum

Pulmonary trunk

Left pulmonary artery

Branches of the
pulmonary veins

Left atrium

Left coronary artery

Circumflex vessels

Anterior interventricular
artery

Great cardiac vein

Left ventricle

Apex of heart

(a)

Anterior View of Heart
Figure 21.2a

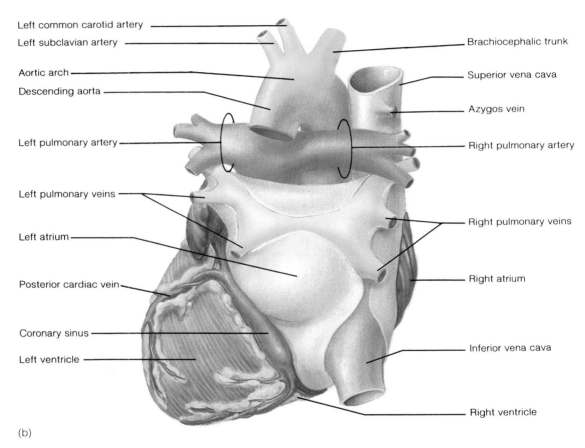

Left common carotid artery

Left subclavian artery

Aortic arch

Descending aorta

Left pulmonary artery

Left pulmonary veins

Left atrium

Posterior cardiac vein

Coronary sinus

Left ventricle

Brachiocephalic trunk

Superior vena cava

Azygos vein

Right pulmonary artery

Right pulmonary veins

Right atrium

Inferior vena cava

Right ventricle

(b)

Posterior View of Heart
Figure 21.2b

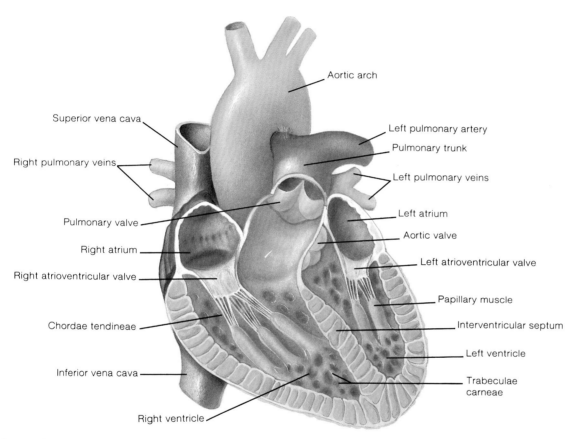

Superior vena cava

Right pulmonary veins

Pulmonary valve

Right atrium

Right atrioventricular valve

Chordae tendineae

Inferior vena cava

Right ventricle

Aortic arch

Left pulmonary artery

Pulmonary trunk

Left pulmonary veins

Left atrium

Aortic valve

Left atrioventricular valve

Papillary muscle

Interventricular septum

Left ventricle

Trabeculae carneae

Internal View of Heart
Figure 21.2c

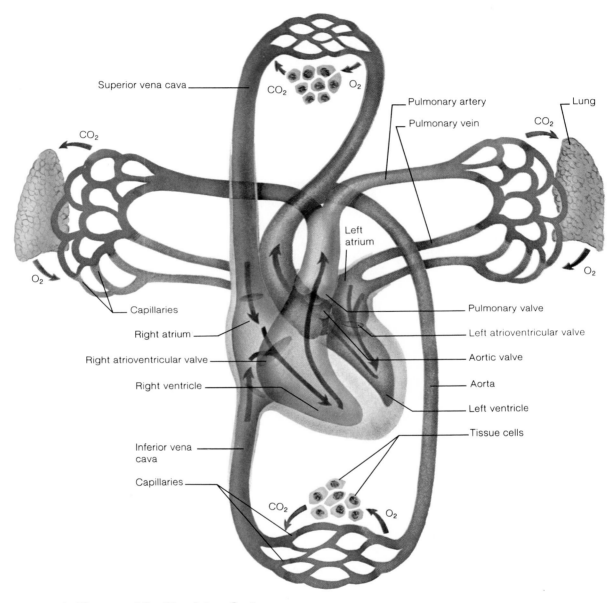

Schematic Diagram of the Circulatory System
Figure 21.3

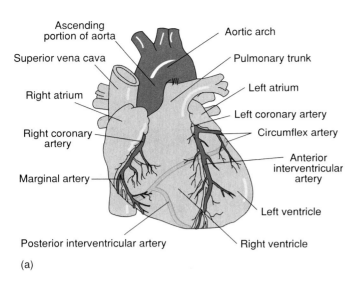

Ascending portion of aorta

Superior vena cava

Right atrium

Right coronary artery

Marginal artery

Posterior interventricular artery

Aortic arch

Pulmonary trunk

Left atrium

Left coronary artery

Circumflex artery

Anterior interventricular artery

Left ventricle

Right ventricle

(a)

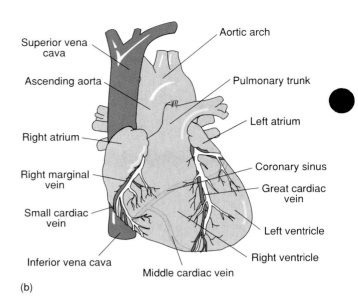

Superior vena cava

Ascending aorta

Right atrium

Right marginal vein

Small cardiac vein

Inferior vena cava

Aortic arch

Pulmonary trunk

Left atrium

Coronary sinus

Great cardiac vein

Left ventricle

Right ventricle

Middle cardiac vein

(b)

Coronary Circulation
Figure 21.5

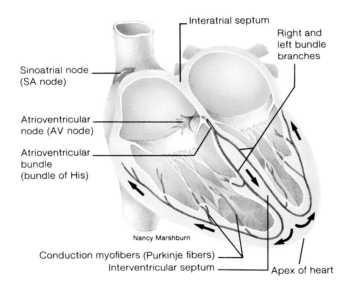

Interatrial septum

Right and left bundle branches

Sinoatrial node (SA node)

Atrioventricular node (AV node)

Atrioventricular bundle (bundle of His)

Nancy Marshburn

Conduction myofibers (Purkinje fibers)

Interventricular septum

Apex of heart

Conduction System of Heart
Figure 21.10

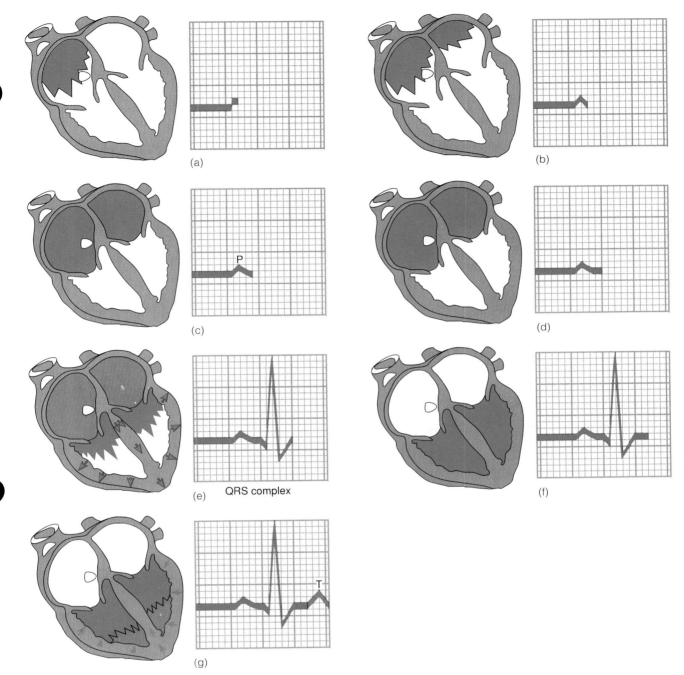

(a)

(b)

(c)

(d)

(e) QRS complex

(f)

(g)

Conduction System of Heart and ECG
Figure 21.13

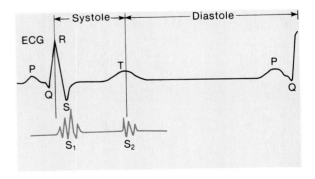

Relationship between the Heart Sounds and the ECG
Figure 21.14

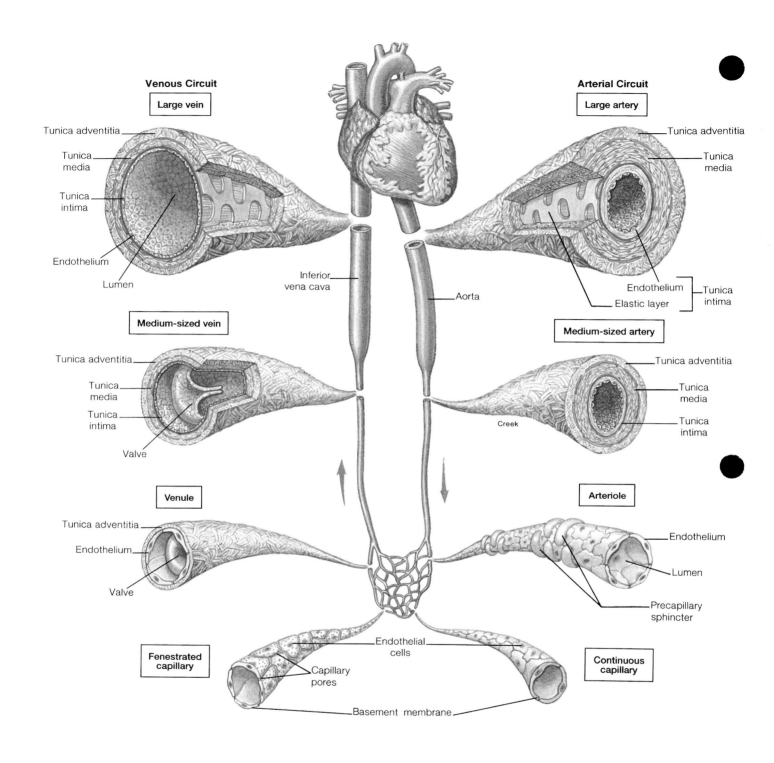

Venous Circuit

Large vein

Tunica adventitia

Tunica media

Tunica intima

Endothelium

Lumen

Inferior vena cava

Medium-sized vein

Tunica adventitia

Tunica media

Tunica intima

Valve

Venule

Tunica adventitia

Endothelium

Valve

Fenestrated capillary

Endothelial cells

Capillary pores

Basement membrane

Arterial Circuit

Large artery

Tunica adventitia

Tunica media

Endothelium

Elastic layer

Tunica intima

Aorta

Medium-sized artery

Tunica adventitia

Tunica media

Tunica intima

Creek

Arteriole

Endothelium

Lumen

Precapillary sphincter

Continuous capillary

Structure of a Medium-sized Artery and Vein
Figure 21.15

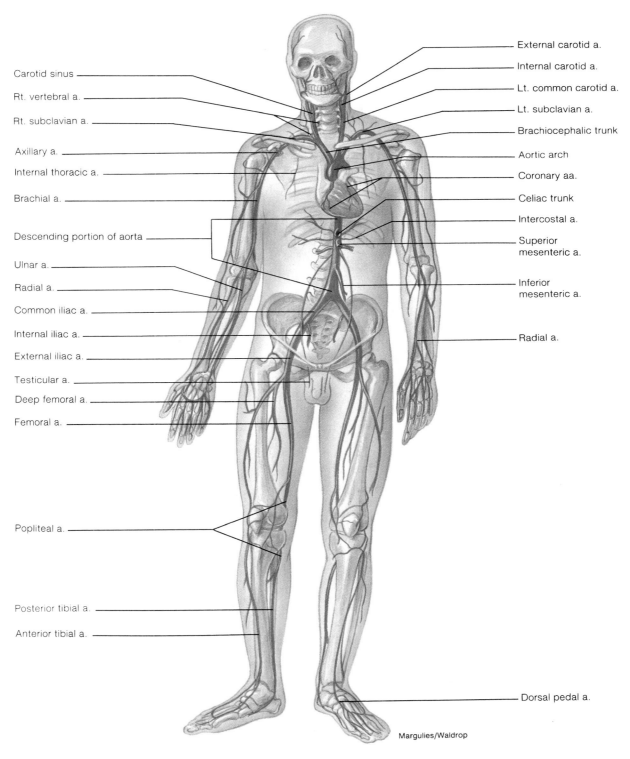

Carotid sinus

Rt. vertebral a.

Rt. subclavian a.

Axillary a.

Internal thoracic a.

Brachial a.

Descending portion of aorta

Ulnar a.

Radial a.

Common iliac a.

Internal iliac a.

External iliac a.

Testicular a.

Deep femoral a.

Femoral a.

Popliteal a.

Posterior tibial a.

Anterior tibial a.

External carotid a.

Internal carotid a.

Lt. common carotid a.

Lt. subclavian a.

Brachiocephalic trunk

Aortic arch

Coronary aa.

Celiac trunk

Intercostal a.

Superior mesenteric a.

Inferior mesenteric a.

Radial a.

Dorsal pedal a.

Margulies/Waldrop

Principal Arteries of Body
Figure 21.19

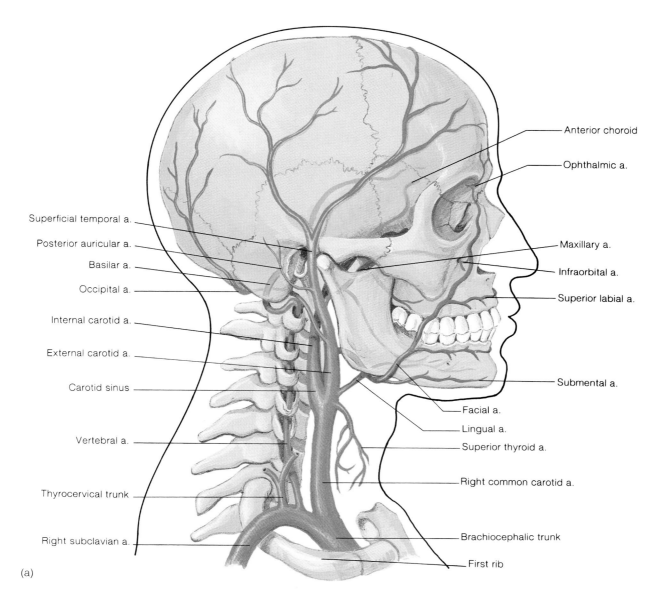

(a)

Anterior choroid

Ophthalmic a.

Superficial temporal a.

Posterior auricular a.

Basilar a.

Occipital a.

Internal carotid a.

External carotid a.

Carotid sinus

Vertebral a.

Thyrocervical trunk

Right subclavian a.

Maxillary a.

Infraorbital a.

Superior labial a.

Submental a.

Facial a.

Lingual a.

Superior thyroid a.

Right common carotid a.

Brachiocephalic trunk

First rib

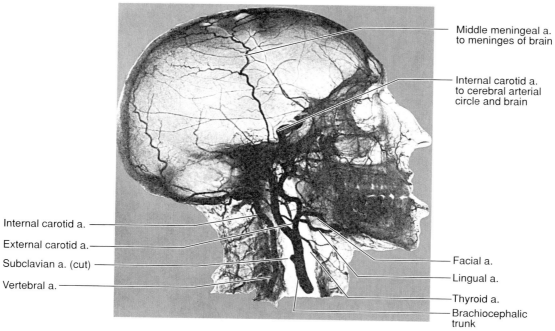

(b)

Middle meningeal a.
to meninges of brain

Internal carotid a.
to cerebral arterial
circle and brain

Internal carotid a.

External carotid a.

Subclavian a. (cut)

Vertebral a.

Facial a.

Lingual a.

Thyroid a.

Brachiocephalic
trunk

Arteries of Neck and Head
Figure 21.21

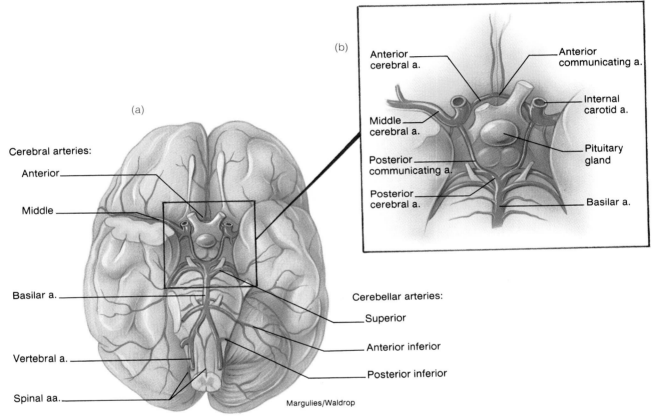

(a)

(b)

Anterior
cerebral a.

Anterior
communicating a.

Middle
cerebral a.

Internal
carotid a.

Posterior
communicating a.

Pituitary
gland

Posterior
cerebral a.

Basilar a.

Cerebral arteries:

Anterior

Middle

Basilar a.

Vertebral a.

Spinal aa.

Cerebellar arteries:

Superior

Anterior inferior

Posterior inferior

Margulies/Waldrop

Arteries to the Brain
Figure 21.22

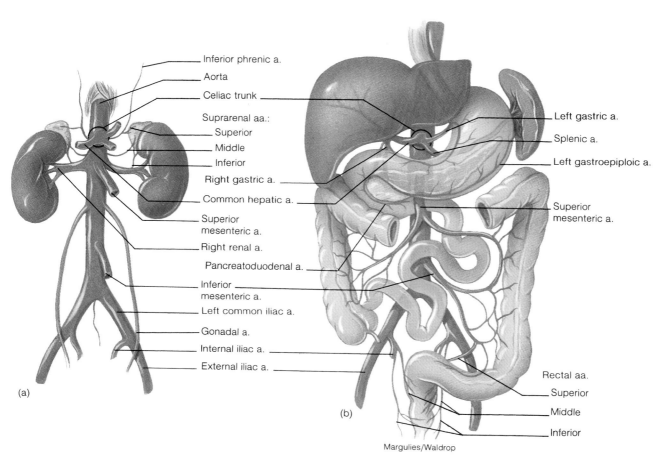

Inferior phrenic a.
Aorta
Celiac trunk
Suprarenal aa.:
  Superior
  Middle
  Inferior
Right gastric a.
Common hepatic a.
Superior mesenteric a.
Right renal a.
Pancreatoduodenal a.
Inferior mesenteric a.
Left common iliac a.
Gonadal a.
Internal iliac a.
External iliac a.

Left gastric a.
Splenic a.
Left gastroepiploic a.
Superior mesenteric a.
Rectal aa.
  Superior
  Middle
  Inferior

(a)

(b)

Margulies/Waldrop

Abdominal Aorta and Principal Branches
Figure 21.26

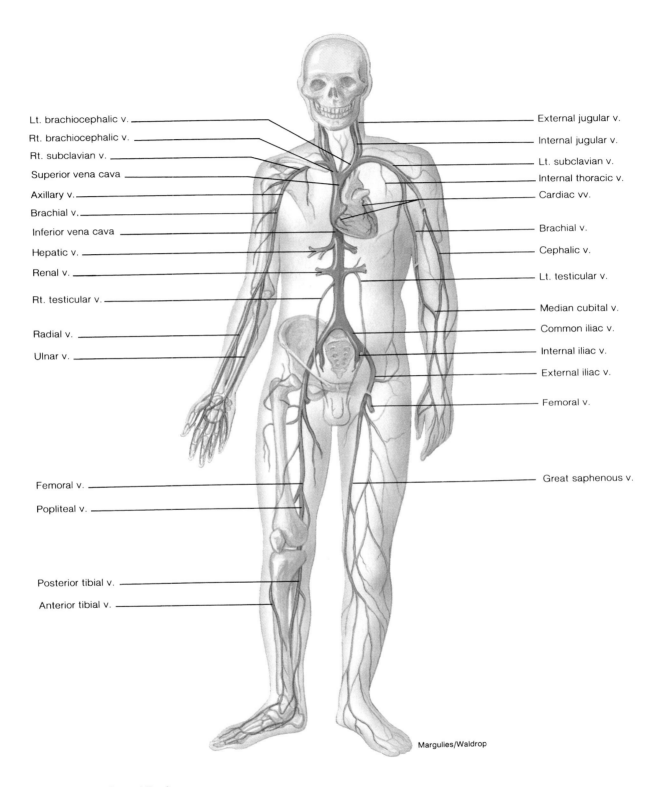

Lt. brachiocephalic v.
Rt. brachiocephalic v.
Rt. subclavian v.
Superior vena cava
Axillary v.
Brachial v.
Inferior vena cava
Hepatic v.
Renal v.
Rt. testicular v.
Radial v.
Ulnar v.

External jugular v.
Internal jugular v.
Lt. subclavian v.
Internal thoracic v.
Cardiac vv.
Brachial v.
Cephalic v.
Lt. testicular v.
Median cubital v.
Common iliac v.
Internal iliac v.
External iliac v.
Femoral v.

Femoral v.
Popliteal v.

Great saphenous v.

Posterior tibial v.
Anterior tibial v.

Margulies/Waldrop

Principal Veins of Body
Figure 21.30

111

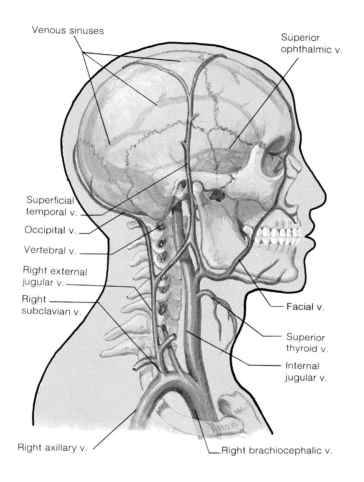

Veins of the Head and Neck
Figure 21.31

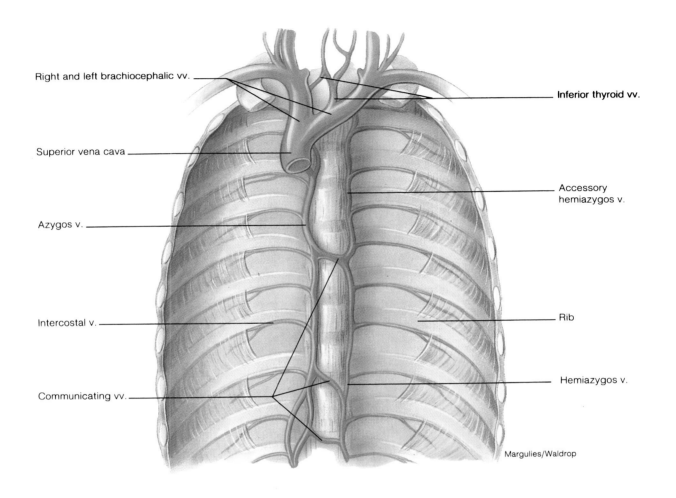

Right and left brachiocephalic vv. ⎯

Inferior thyroid vv.

Superior vena cava ⎯

Accessory hemiazygos v.

Azygos v. ⎯

Intercostal v. ⎯

Rib

Hemiazygos v.

Communicating vv. ⎯

Margulies/Waldrop

Veins of the Thoracic Region
Figure 21.34

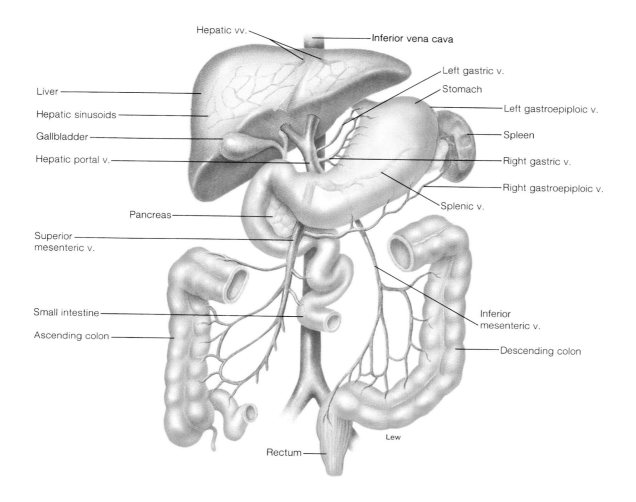

Hepatic vv.

Inferior vena cava

Left gastric v.

Stomach

Liver

Hepatic sinusoids

Gallbladder

Hepatic portal v.

Left gastroepiploic v.

Spleen

Right gastric v.

Right gastroepiploic v.

Splenic v.

Pancreas

Superior
mesenteric v.

Small intestine

Ascending colon

Inferior
mesenteric v.

Descending colon

Rectum

Lew

Hepatic Portal System
Figure 21.36

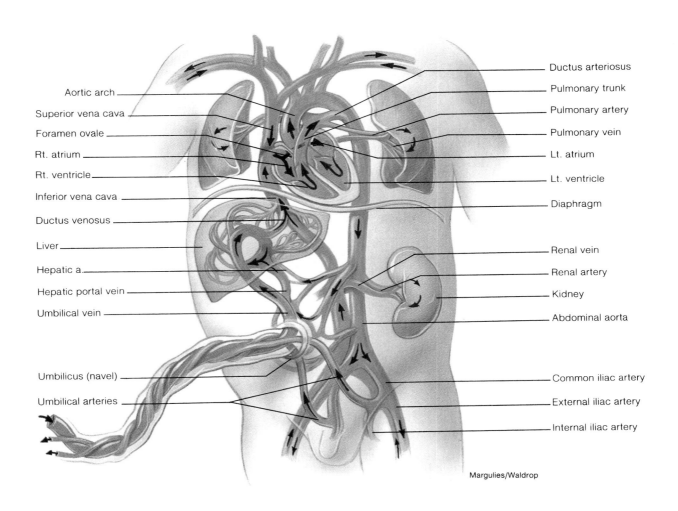

Aortic arch

Superior vena cava

Foramen ovale

Rt. atrium

Rt. ventricle

Inferior vena cava

Ductus venosus

Liver

Hepatic a.

Hepatic portal vein

Umbilical vein

Umbilicus (navel)

Umbilical arteries

Ductus arteriosus

Pulmonary trunk

Pulmonary artery

Pulmonary vein

Lt. atrium

Lt. ventricle

Diaphragm

Renal vein

Renal artery

Kidney

Abdominal aorta

Common iliac artery

External iliac artery

Internal iliac artery

Margulies/Waldrop

Fetal Circulation
Figure 21.37

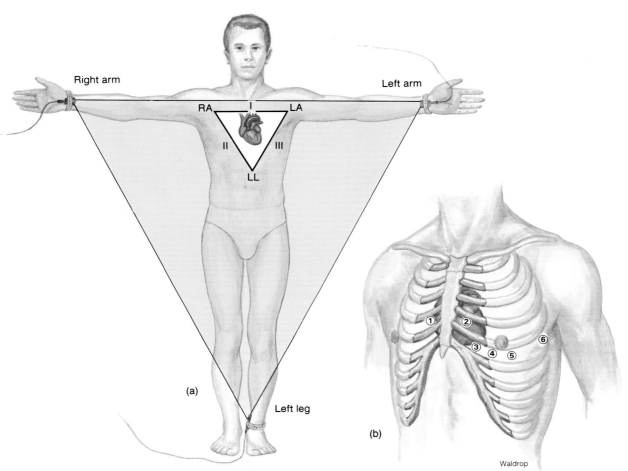

Right arm

Left arm

RA   I   LA

II   III

LL

(a)

Left leg

(b)

① ② ③ ④ ⑤ ⑥

Waldrop

Placement of Bipolar Limb Leads
Figure 21.38

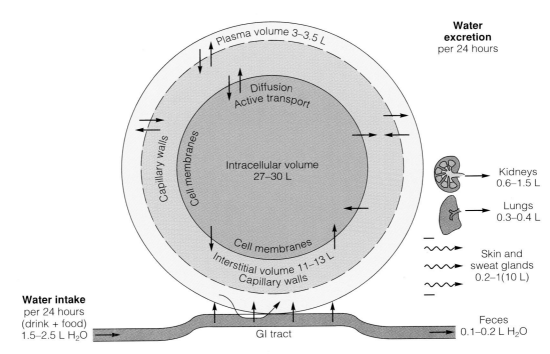

Daily Intake and Excretion of Body Water
Figure 22.6

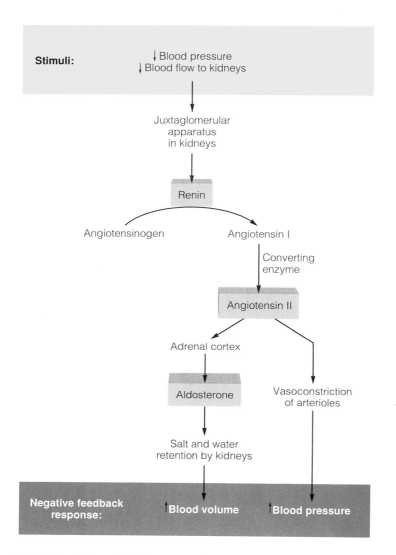

Renin-Angiotensin-Aldosterone System
Figure 22.11

118

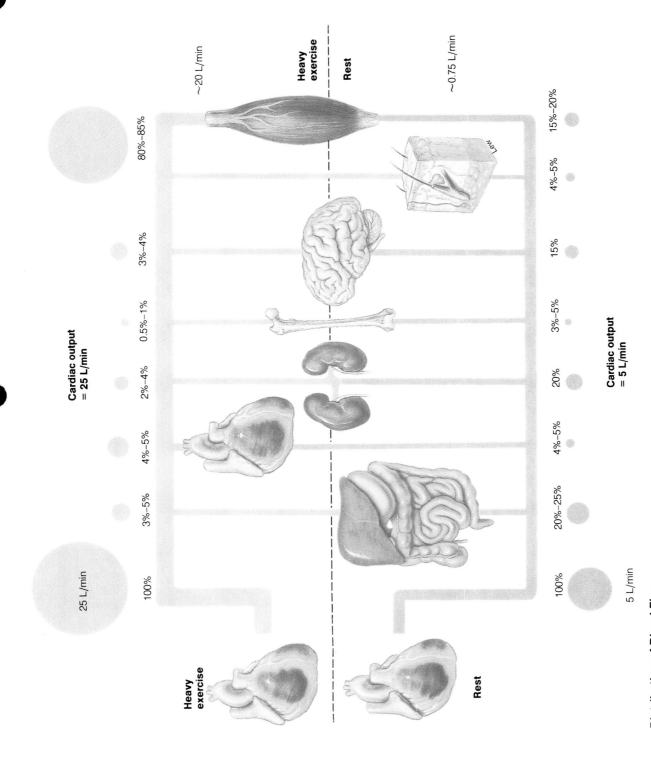

Distribution of Blood Flow
Figure 22.17

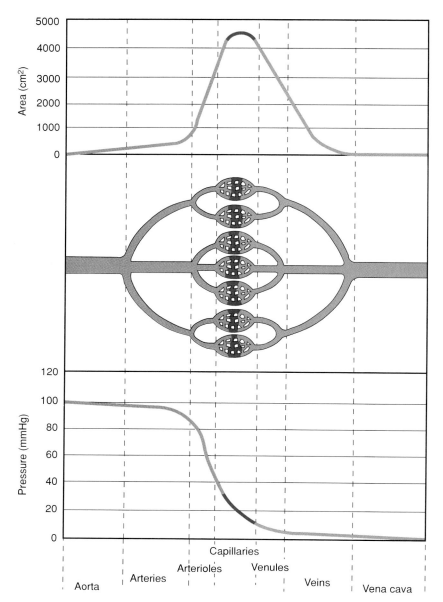

Relationship between Cross-Sectional Area and Pressure in Blood Vessels
Figure 22.22

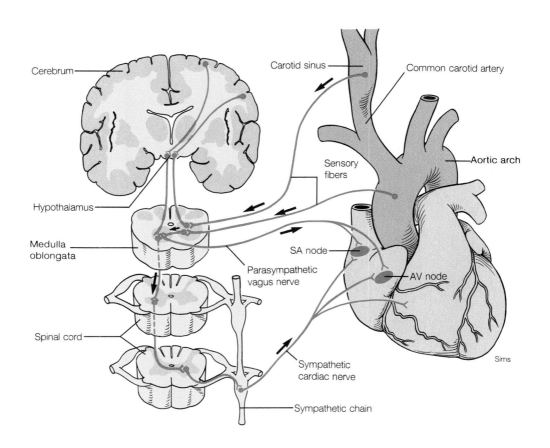

Cerebrum

Carotid sinus

Common carotid artery

Aortic arch

Sensory fibers

Hypothalamus

Medulla oblongata

SA node

Parasympathetic vagus nerve

AV node

Spinal cord

Sympathetic cardiac nerve

Sympathetic chain

Sims

Baroreceptor Reflex
Figure 22.23

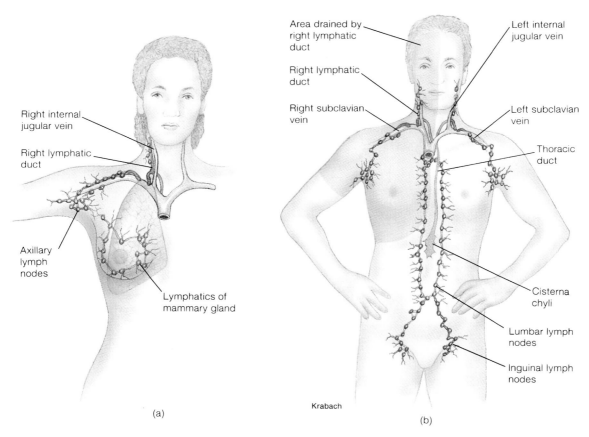

(a)

Right internal jugular vein

Right lymphatic duct

Axillary lymph nodes

Lymphatics of mammary gland

Area drained by right lymphatic duct

Right lymphatic duct

Right subclavian vein

Left internal jugular vein

Left subclavian vein

Thoracic duct

Cisterna chyli

Lumbar lymph nodes

Inguinal lymph nodes

Krabach

(b)

Lymphatic Vessels
Figure 23.1

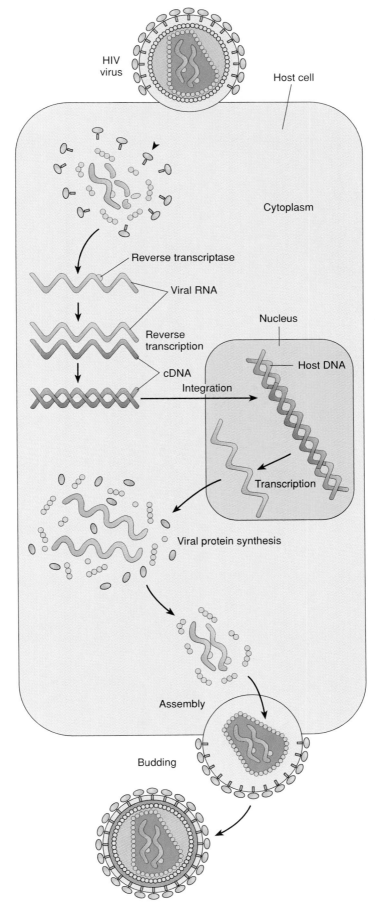

Labels within the figure:

HIV virus

Host cell

Cytoplasm

Reverse transcriptase

Viral RNA

Reverse transcription

cDNA

Integration

Nucleus

Host DNA

Transcription

Viral protein synthesis

Assembly

Budding

Life Cycle of the Human Immunodeficiency Virus (HIV)
Figure 23.8

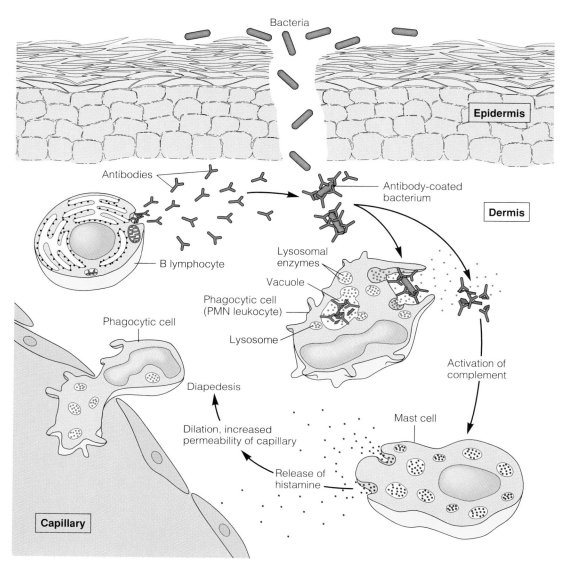

Bacteria

Epidermis

Antibodies

Antibody-coated
bacterium

Dermis

B lymphocyte

Lysosomal
enzymes

Vacuole

Phagocytic cell
(PMN leukocyte)

Lysosome

Activation of
complement

Phagocytic cell

Diapedesis

Mast cell

Dilation, increased
permeability of capillary

Release of
histamine

Capillary

A Local Inflammatory Reaction
Figure 23.16

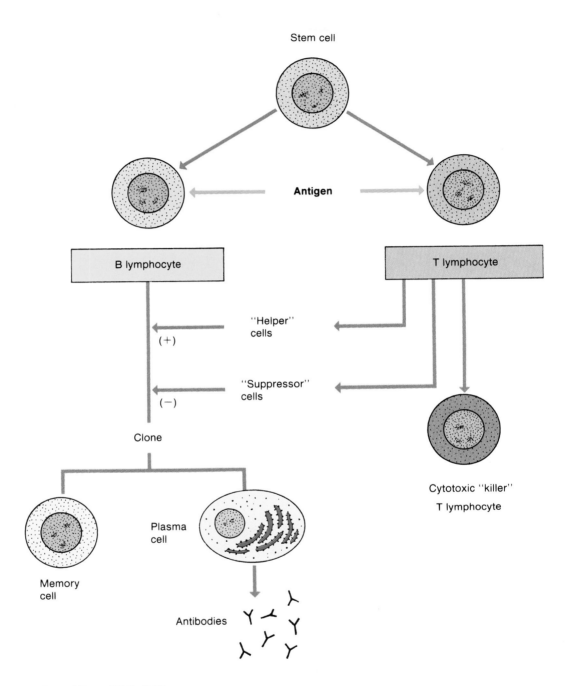

Stem cell

Antigen

B lymphocyte

T lymphocyte

"Helper" cells

(+)

"Suppressor" cells

(−)

Clone

Memory cell

Plasma cell

Antibodies

Cytotoxic "killer" T lymphocyte

Stimulation of B and T Cell Clones
Figure 23.21

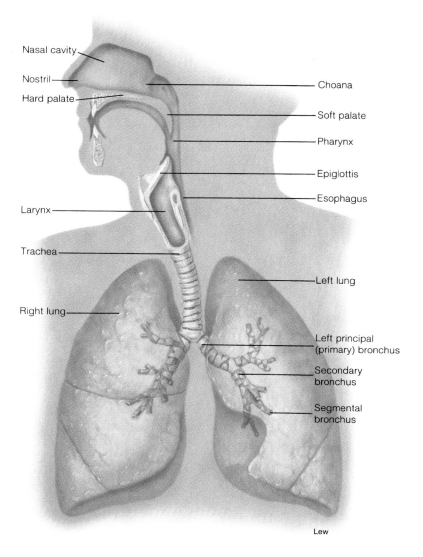

Nasal cavity
Nostril
Hard palate
Larynx
Trachea
Right lung
Choana
Soft palate
Pharynx
Epiglottis
Esophagus
Left lung
Left principal
(primary) bronchus
Secondary
bronchus
Segmental
bronchus

Lew

Anatomy of Respiratory System
Figure 24.1

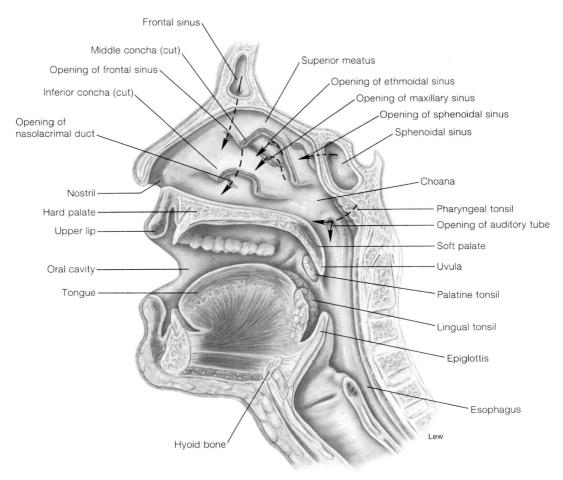

Frontal sinus

Middle concha (cut)

Opening of frontal sinus

Inferior concha (cut)

Opening of
nasolacrimal duct

Nostril

Hard palate

Upper lip

Oral cavity

Tongue

Hyoid bone

Superior meatus

Opening of ethmoidal sinus

Opening of maxillary sinus

Opening of sphenoidal sinus

Sphenoidal sinus

Choana

Pharyngeal tonsil

Opening of auditory tube

Soft palate

Uvula

Palatine tonsil

Lingual tonsil

Epiglottis

Esophagus

Lew

Structures of Upper Respiratory Tract
Figure 24.2

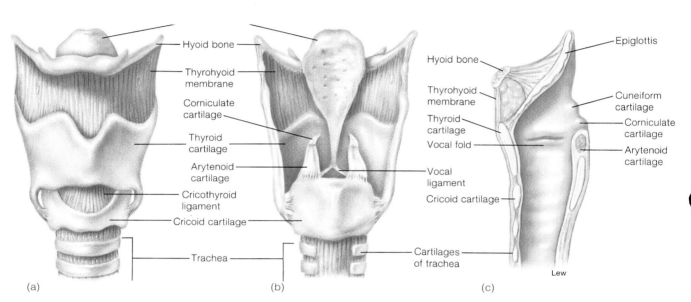

Hyoid bone

Thyrohyoid membrane

Corniculate cartilage

Thyroid cartilage

Arytenoid cartilage

Cricothyroid ligament

Cricoid cartilage

Trachea

(a)

Vocal ligament

Cartilages of trachea

(b)

Hyoid bone

Thyrohyoid membrane

Thyroid cartilage

Vocal fold

Cricoid cartilage

Epiglottis

Cuneiform cartilage

Corniculate cartilage

Arytenoid cartilage

Lew

(c)

Structure of Larynx
Figure 24.5

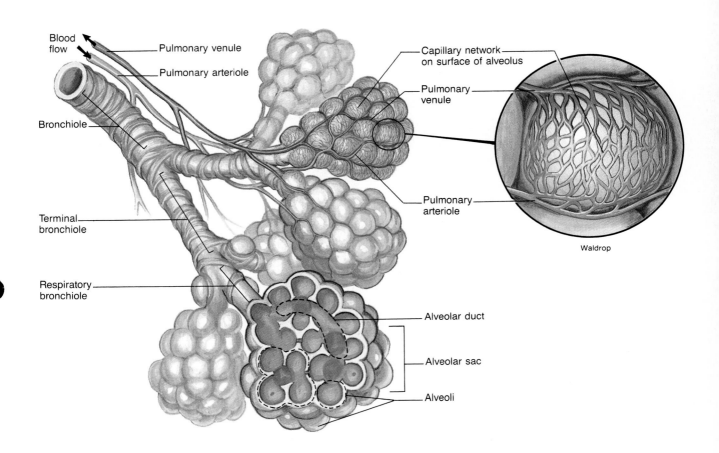

Blood flow

Pulmonary venule

Pulmonary arteriole

Bronchiole

Terminal bronchiole

Respiratory bronchiole

Capillary network on surface of alveolus

Pulmonary venule

Pulmonary arteriole

Waldrop

Alveolar duct

Alveolar sac

Alveoli

Pulmonary Capillaries and Alveoli
Figure 24.9

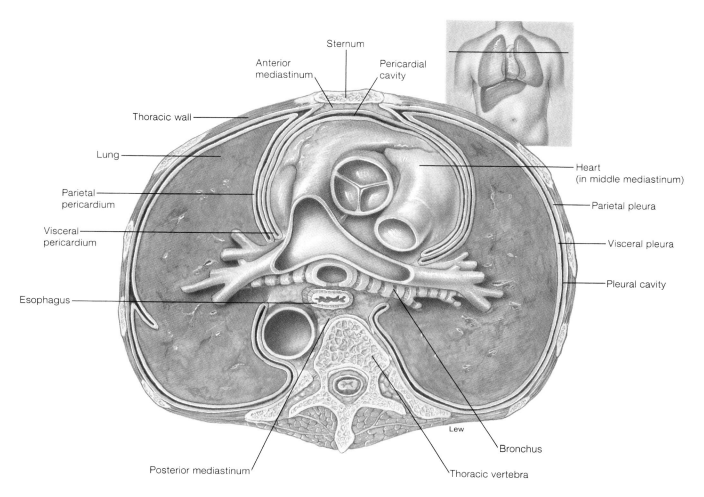

Sternum

Anterior mediastinum

Pericardial cavity

Thoracic wall

Lung

Parietal pericardium

Visceral pericardium

Esophagus

Heart (in middle mediastinum)

Parietal pleura

Visceral pleura

Pleural cavity

Lew

Posterior mediastinum

Bronchus

Thoracic vertebra

Cross Section of Thoracic Cavity
Figure 24.12

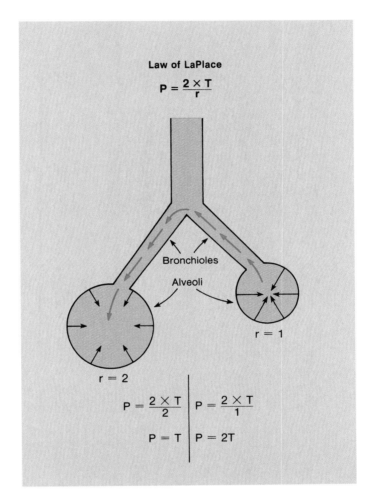

Law of LaPlace
Figure 24.16

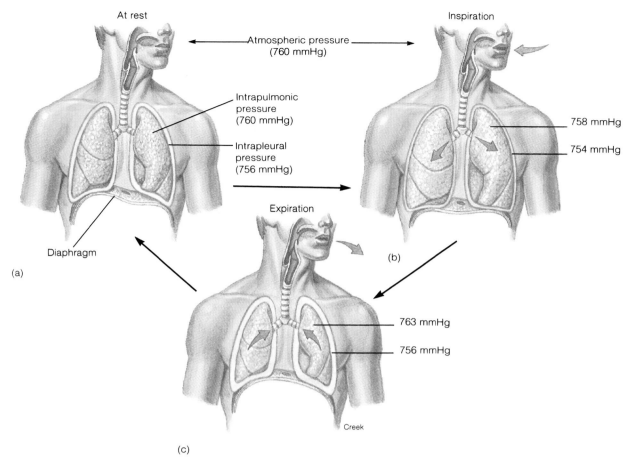

At rest

Atmospheric pressure
(760 mmHg)

Inspiration

Intrapulmonic
pressure
(760 mmHg)

Intrapleural
pressure
(756 mmHg)

758 mmHg

754 mmHg

Diaphragm

(a)

(b)

Expiration

763 mmHg

756 mmHg

Creek

(c)

Pulmonary Ventilation
Figure 24.20

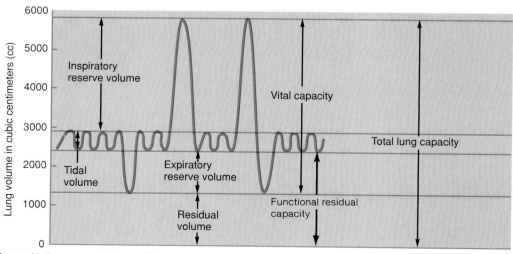

Lung Volumes and Capacities
Figure 24.22

Lung volume in cubic centimeters (cc)

Inspiratory
reserve volume

Vital capacity

Total lung capacity

Tidal
volume

Expiratory
reserve volume

Functional residual
capacity

Residual
volume

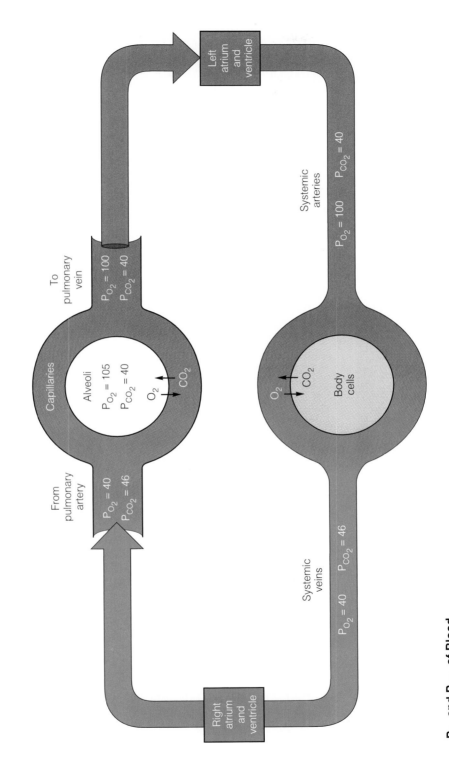

P$_{O_2}$ and P$_{CO_2}$ of Blood
Figure 24.27

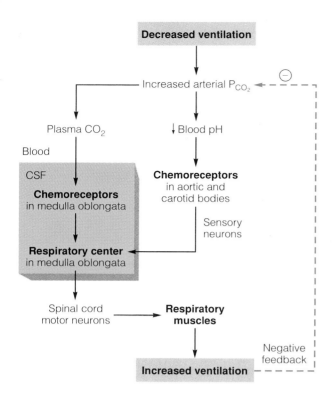

Negative Feedback Control of Ventilation
Figure 24.31

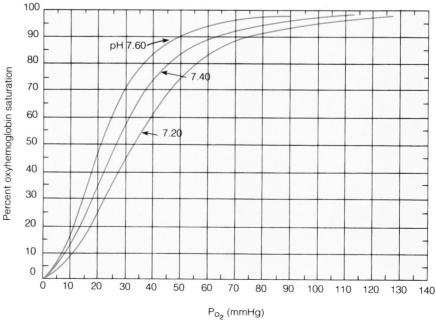

Oxyhemoglobin Dissociation Curve
Figure 24.36

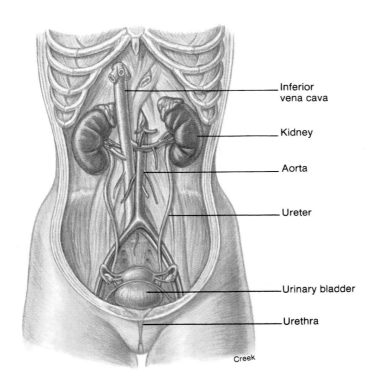

Inferior vena cava

Kidney

Aorta

Ureter

Urinary bladder

Urethra

Creek

Basic Anatomy of Urinary System
Figure 25.1

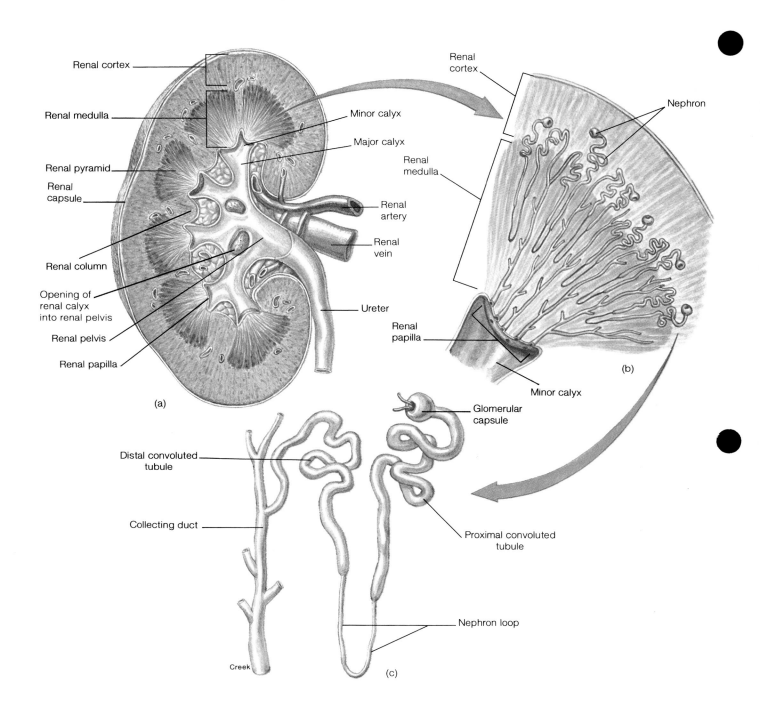

(a)

Renal cortex

Renal medulla

Renal pyramid

Renal capsule

Renal column

Opening of renal calyx into renal pelvis

Renal pelvis

Renal papilla

Minor calyx

Major calyx

Renal artery

Renal vein

Ureter

Renal cortex

Nephron

Renal medulla

Renal papilla

Minor calyx

(b)

Distal convoluted tubule

Collecting duct

Creek

Glomerular capsule

Proximal convoluted tubule

Nephron loop

(c)

Structure of Kidney
Figure 25.3

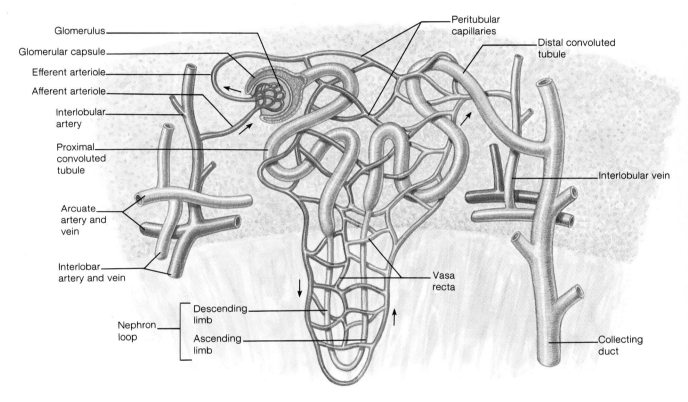

Glomerulus

Glomerular capsule

Efferent arteriole

Afferent arteriole

Interlobular artery

Proximal convoluted tubule

Arcuate artery and vein

Interlobar artery and vein

Nephron loop

Descending limb

Ascending limb

Peritubular capillaries

Distal convoluted tubule

Interlobular vein

Vasa recta

Collecting duct

Blood Flow in Association with the Nephron
Figure 25.5

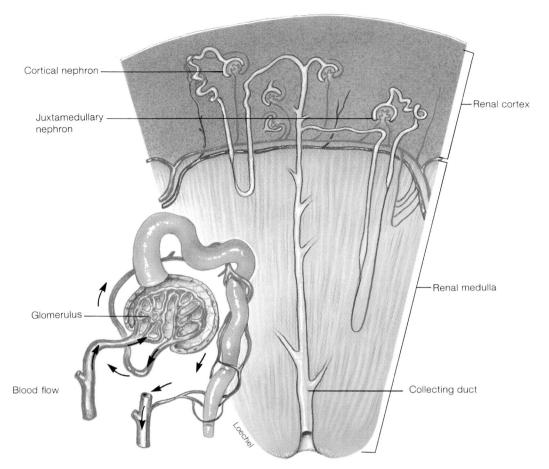

Cortical and Juxtamedullary Nephrons within the Kidney
Figure 25.6

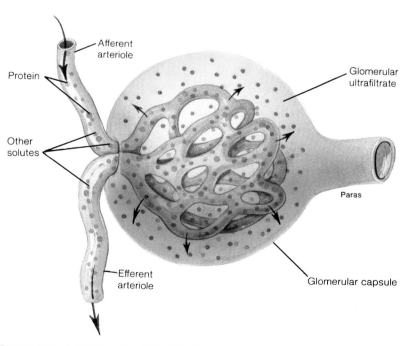

Formation of Glomerular Ultrafiltrate
Figure 25.10

138

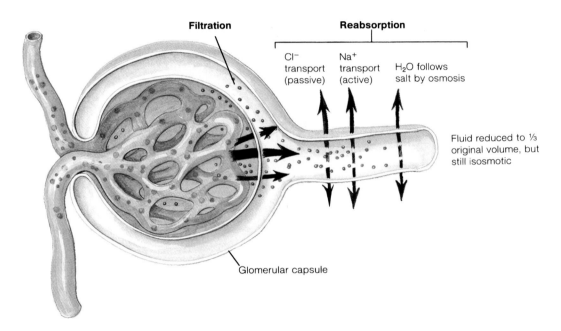

Filtration

Reabsorption

Cl⁻
transport
(passive)

Na⁺
transport
(active)

H_2O follows
salt by osmosis

Fluid reduced to ⅓
original volume, but
still isosmotic

Glomerular capsule

Mechanisms of Salt and Water Reabsorption in the Proximal Convoluted Tubule
Figure 25.14

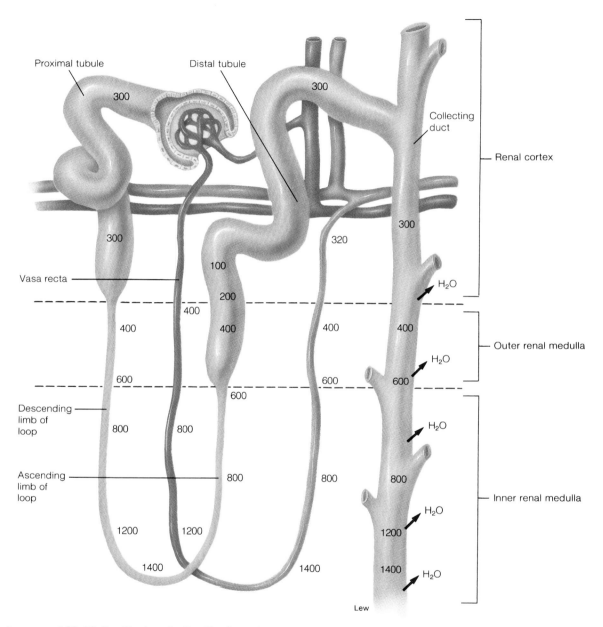

Countercurrent Multiplier System in the Nephron Loop
Figure 25.19

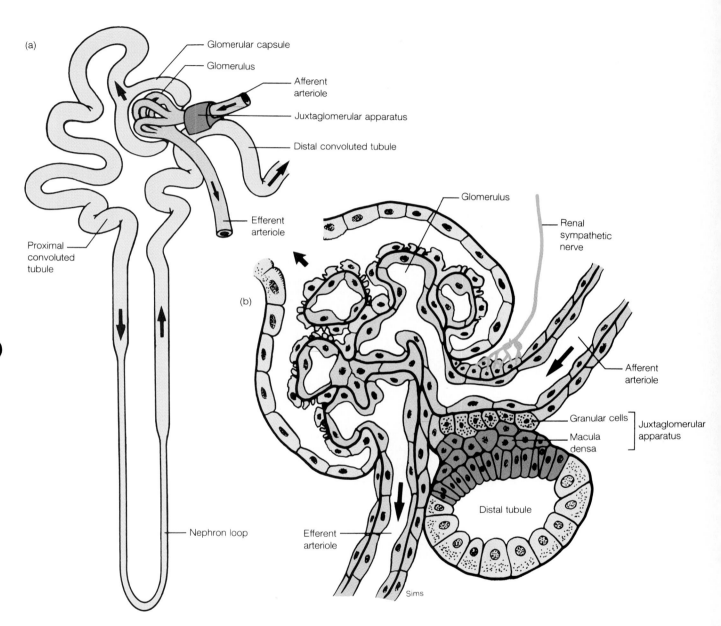

(a)

Glomerular capsule

Glomerulus

Afferent arteriole

Juxtaglomerular apparatus

Distal convoluted tubule

Efferent arteriole

Proximal convoluted tubule

Nephron loop

(b)

Glomerulus

Renal sympathetic nerve

Afferent arteriole

Granular cells

Macula densa

Juxtaglomerular apparatus

Distal tubule

Efferent arteriole

Sims

Juxtaglomerular Apparatus
Figure 25.24

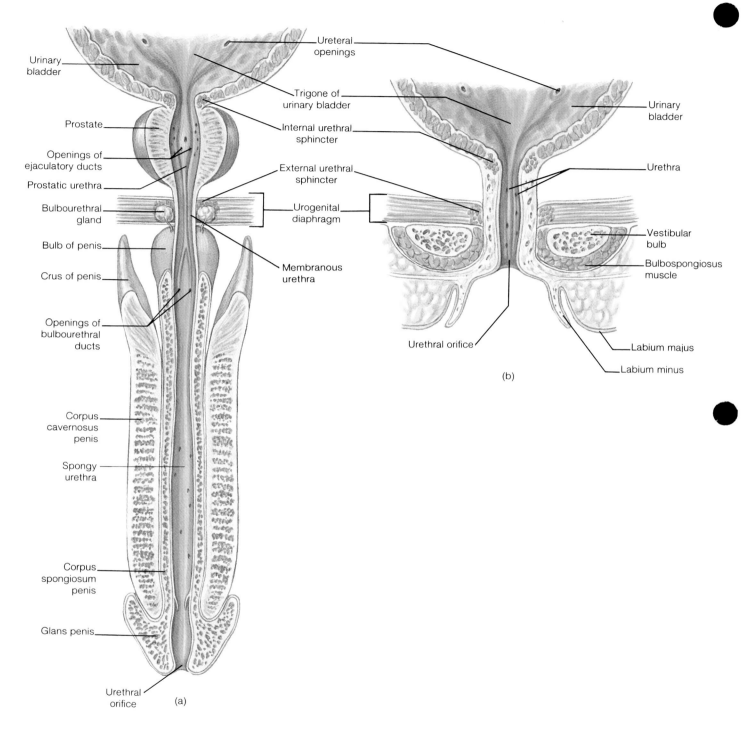

Urinary bladder

Ureteral openings

Trigone of urinary bladder

Internal urethral sphincter

Prostate

Openings of ejaculatory ducts

Prostatic urethra

External urethral sphincter

Bulbourethral gland

Urogenital diaphragm

Bulb of penis

Crus of penis

Membranous urethra

Openings of bulbourethral ducts

Corpus cavernosus penis

Spongy urethra

Corpus spongiosum penis

Glans penis

Urethral orifice

(a)

Urinary bladder

Urethra

Vestibular bulb

Bulbospongiosus muscle

Urethral orifice

Labium majus

Labium minus

(b)

Urinary Bladder and Urethra
Figure 25.29

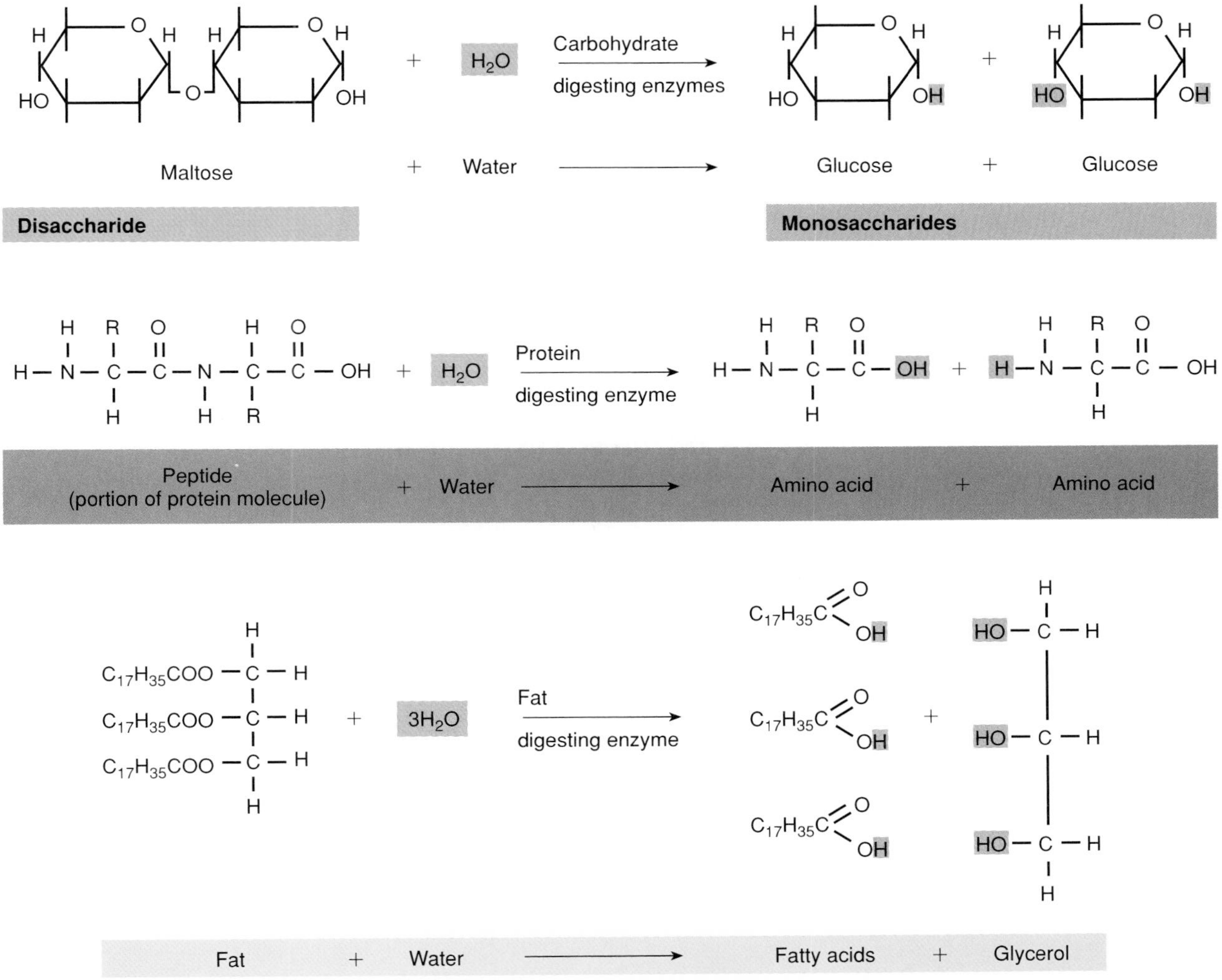

Digestion of Food Molecules by Hydrolysis Reactions
Figure 26.1

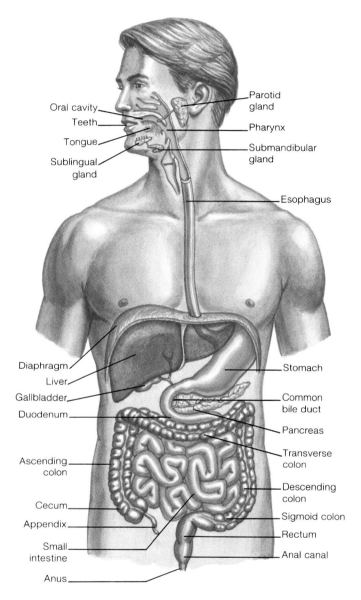

Oral cavity

Teeth

Tongue

Sublingual
gland

Parotid
gland

Pharynx

Submandibular
gland

Esophagus

Diaphragm

Liver

Gallbladder

Duodenum

Ascending
colon

Cecum

Appendix

Small
intestine

Anus

Stomach

Common
bile duct

Pancreas

Transverse
colon

Descending
colon

Sigmoid colon

Rectum

Anal canal

Basic Anatomy of the Digestive System
Figure 26.2

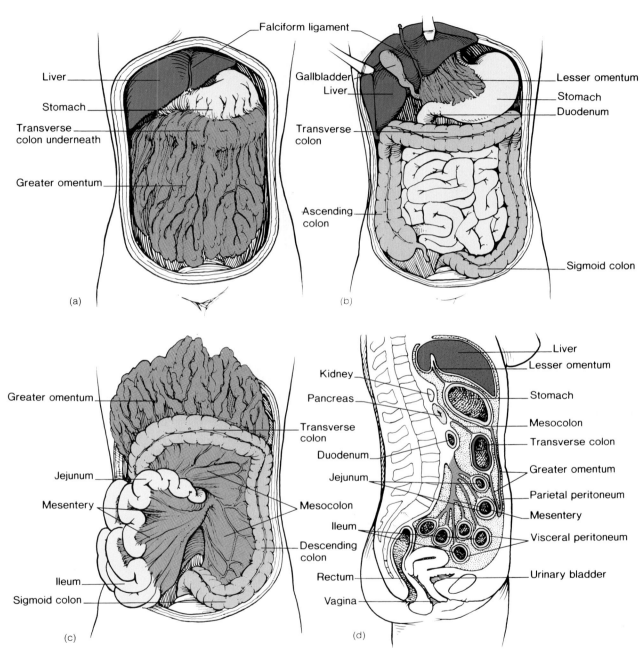

(a)

(b)

Falciform ligament

Liver

Stomach

Transverse colon underneath

Greater omentum

Gallbladder

Liver

Transverse colon

Ascending colon

Lesser omentum

Stomach

Duodenum

Sigmoid colon

(c)

Greater omentum

Jejunum

Mesentery

Ileum

Sigmoid colon

Transverse colon

Mesocolon

Descending colon

(d)

Kidney

Pancreas

Transverse colon

Duodenum

Jejunum

Ileum

Rectum

Vagina

Liver

Lesser omentum

Stomach

Mesocolon

Transverse colon

Greater omentum

Parietal peritoneum

Mesentery

Visceral peritoneum

Urinary bladder

Peritoneal Membranes
Figure 26.4

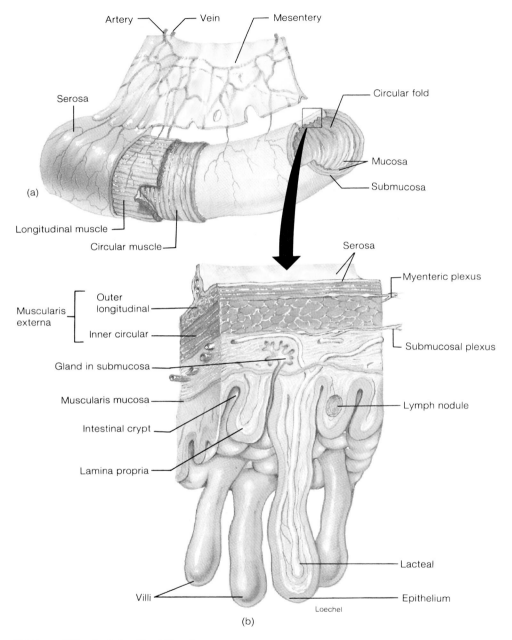

Artery — Vein — Mesentery

Serosa

Circular fold

(a)

Mucosa

Submucosa

Longitudinal muscle

Circular muscle

Serosa

Myenteric plexus

Muscularis externa

Outer longitudinal

Inner circular

Submucosal plexus

Gland in submucosa

Muscularis mucosa

Lymph nodule

Intestinal crypt

Lamina propria

Lacteal

Villi

Epithelium

Loechel

(b)

Tunics of Gastrointestinal Tract
Figure 26.5

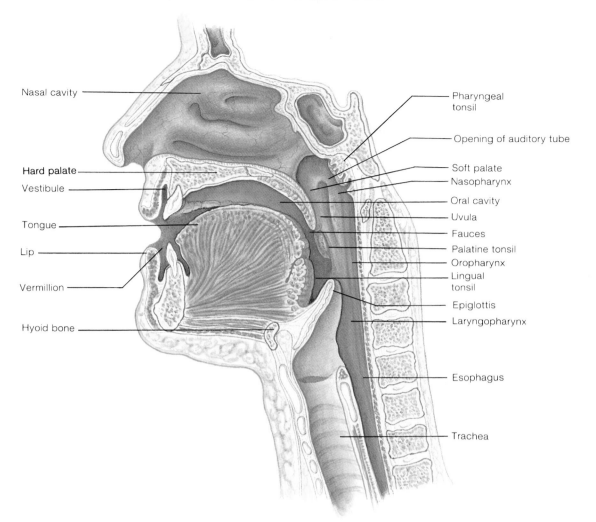

Structure of Oral Cavity and Pharynx
Figure 26.7

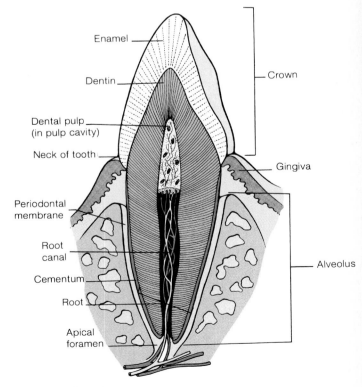

Structure of Tooth
Figure 26.11

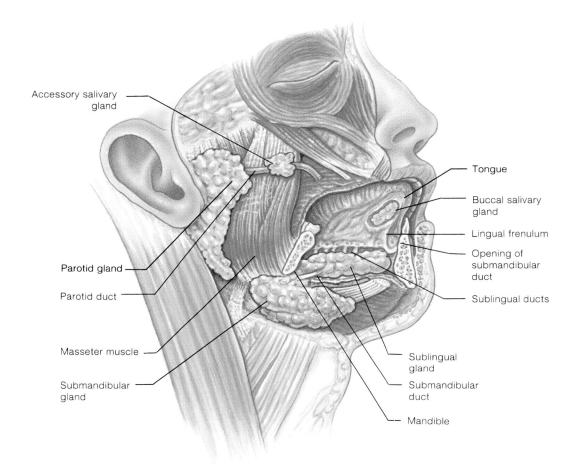

Accessory salivary gland

Tongue

Buccal salivary gland

Parotid gland

Lingual frenulum

Parotid duct

Opening of submandibular duct

Sublingual ducts

Masseter muscle

Sublingual gland

Submandibular gland

Submandibular duct

Mandible

Salivary Glands
Figure 26.12

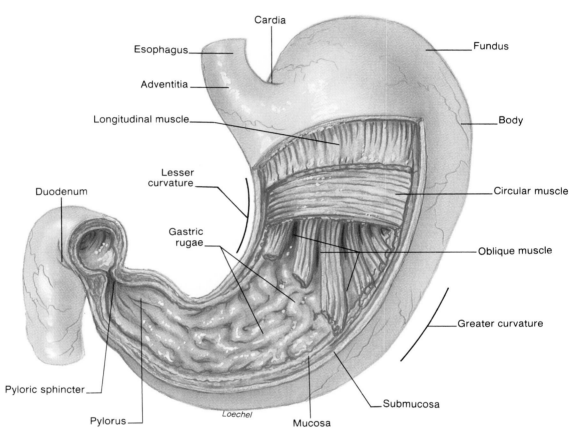

Structure of Stomach
Figure 26.15

Cardia

Esophagus

Adventitia

Longitudinal muscle

Lesser curvature

Duodenum

Gastric rugae

Pyloric sphincter

Pylorus

Loechel

Mucosa

Fundus

Body

Circular muscle

Oblique muscle

Greater curvature

Submucosa

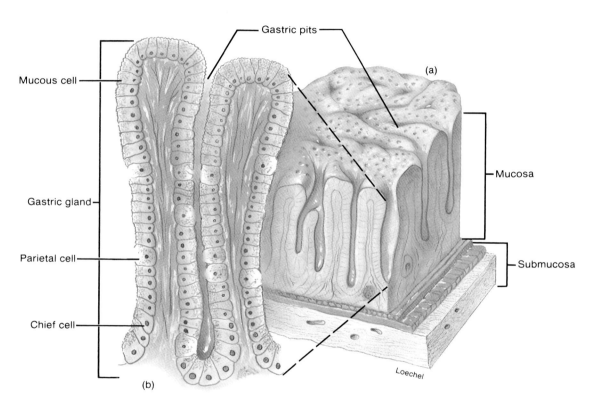

Gastric pits

(a)

Mucous cell

Gastric gland

Parietal cell

Chief cell

Mucosa

Submucosa

Loechel

(b)

Gastric Pits and Gastric Glands of the Mucosa
Figure 26.17

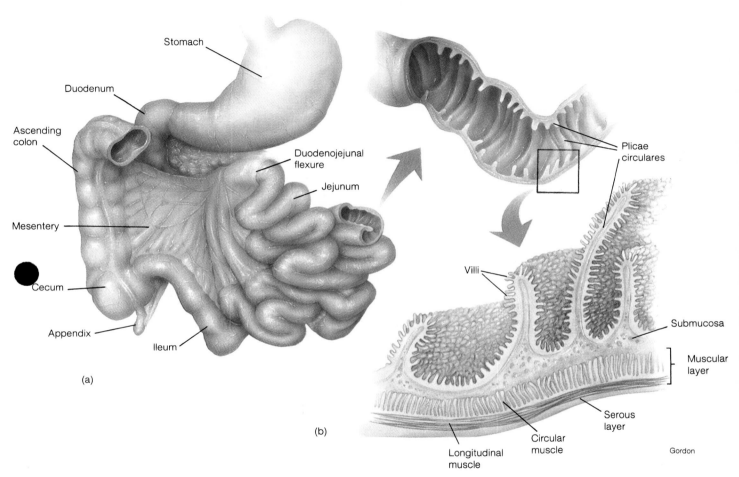

Stomach

Duodenum

Ascending
colon

Mesentery

Cecum

Appendix

Ileum

Duodenojejunal
flexure

Jejunum

(a)

Plicae
circulares

Villi

Submucosa

Muscular
layer

Serous
layer

Circular
muscle

Longitudinal
muscle

Gordon

(b)

Small Intestine
Figure 26.19

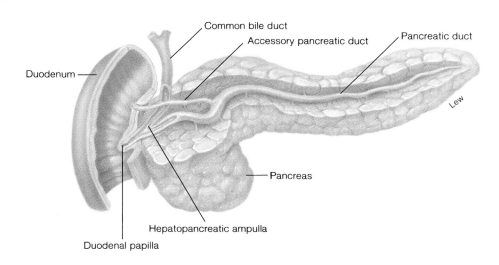

Duodenum and Associated Structures
Figure 26.20

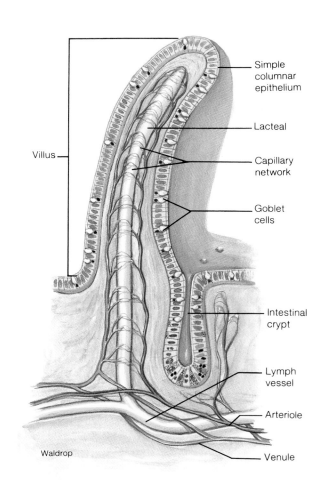

Intestinal Villus
Figure 26.22

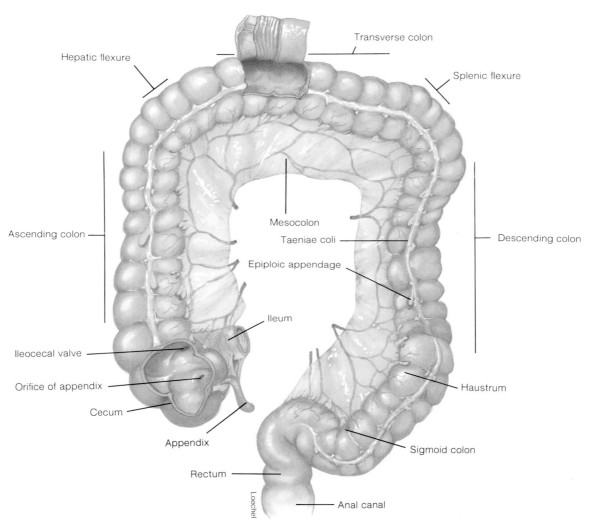

Hepatic flexure

Transverse colon

Splenic flexure

Ascending colon

Mesocolon

Taeniae coli

Epiploic appendage

Descending colon

Ileum

Ileocecal valve

Orifice of appendix

Cecum

Haustrum

Appendix

Sigmoid colon

Rectum

Loechel

Anal canal

Large Intestine
Figure 26.27

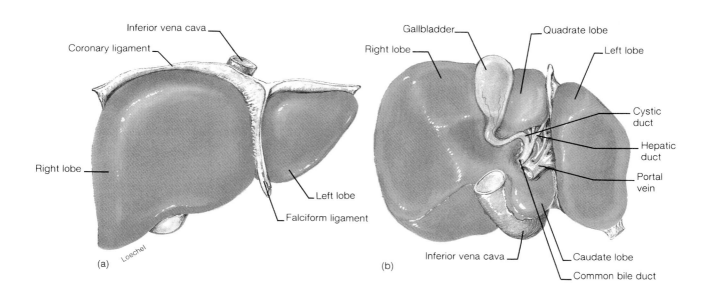

Inferior vena cava

Coronary ligament

Right lobe

Left lobe

Falciform ligament

(a) Loechel

Gallbladder

Quadrate lobe

Right lobe

Left lobe

Cystic duct

Hepatic duct

Portal vein

Inferior vena cava

Caudate lobe

Common bile duct

(b)

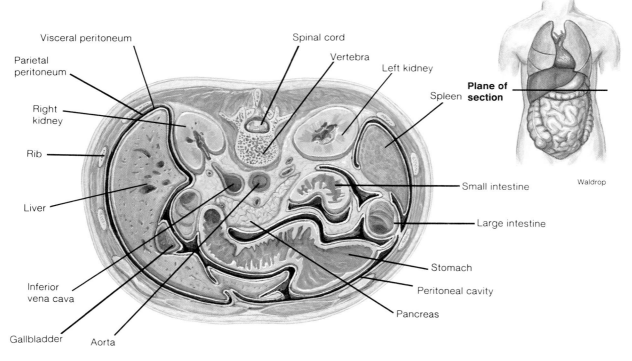

Visceral peritoneum

Spinal cord

Vertebra

Left kidney

Spleen

Plane of section

Parietal peritoneum

Right kidney

Rib

Liver

Inferior vena cava

Gallbladder

Aorta

Small intestine

Large intestine

Stomach

Peritoneal cavity

Pancreas

Waldrop

Liver
Figure 26.30

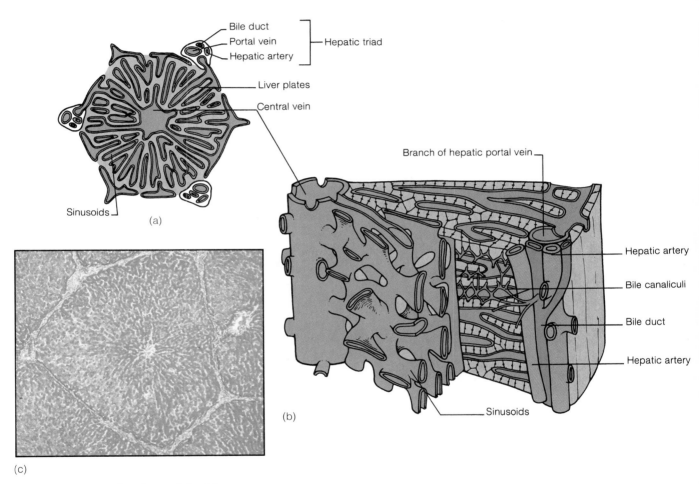

Bile duct
Portal vein — Hepatic triad
Hepatic artery

Liver plates

Central vein

Sinusoids
(a)

Branch of hepatic portal vein

Hepatic artery

Bile canaliculi

Bile duct

Hepatic artery

Sinusoids
(b)

(c)

Liver Lobule and Histology of the Liver
Figure 26.31

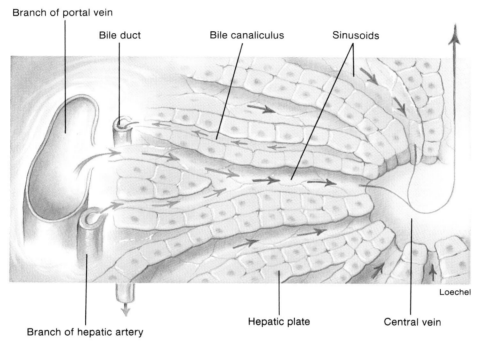

Branch of portal vein

Bile duct

Bile canaliculus

Sinusoids

Loechel

Branch of hepatic artery

Hepatic plate

Central vein

Flow of Blood and Bile in a Liver Lobule
Figure 26.32

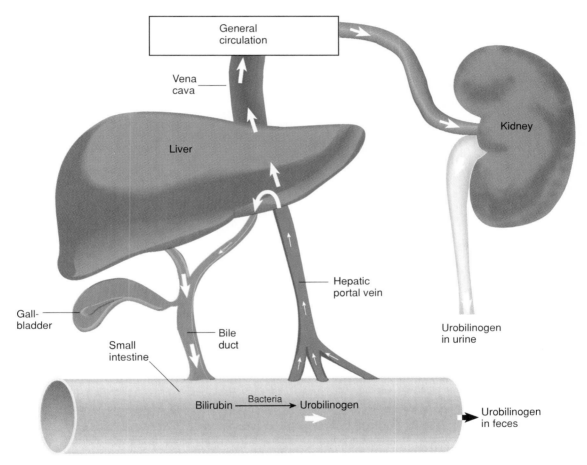

Enterohepatic Circulation of Urobilinogen
Figure 26.34

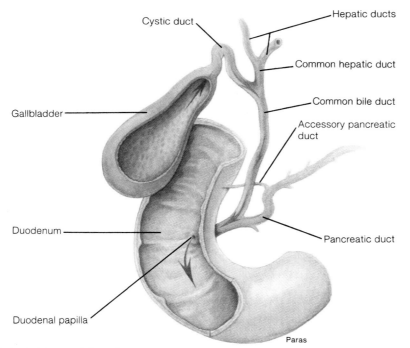

Cystic duct

Hepatic ducts

Common hepatic duct

Common bile duct

Accessory pancreatic
duct

Gallbladder

Duodenum

Pancreatic duct

Duodenal papilla

Paras

Gallbladder and Duodenum
Figure 26.36

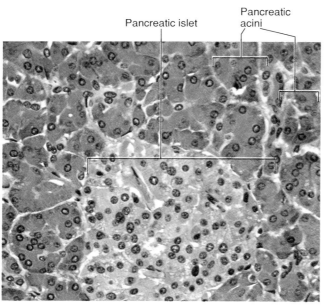

Pancreatic
acini

Pancreatic islet

Pancreatic Islet Cells
Figure 26.38

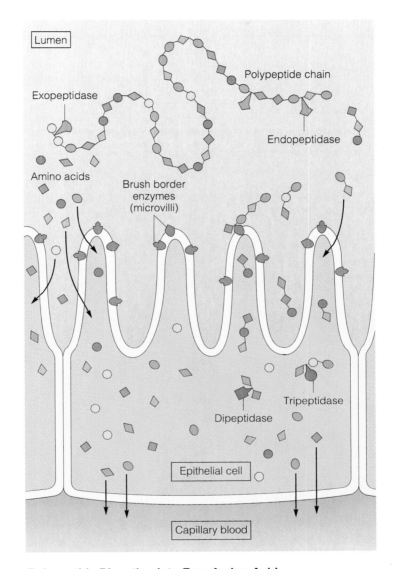

Polypeptide Digestion into Free Amino Acids
Figure 26.41

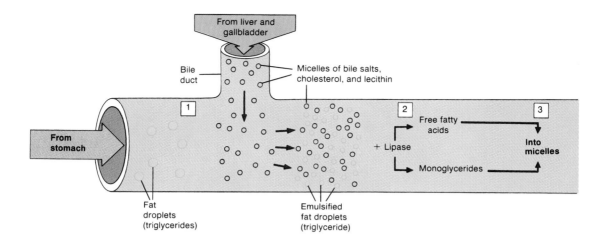

Step 1 Emulsification of fat droplets by bile salts

Step 2 Hydrolysis of triglycerides in emulsified fat droplets into fatty acid and monoglycerides

Step 3 Dissolving of fatty acids and monoglycerides into micelles to produce "mixed micelles"

Steps in the Digestion of Fat
Figure 26.43

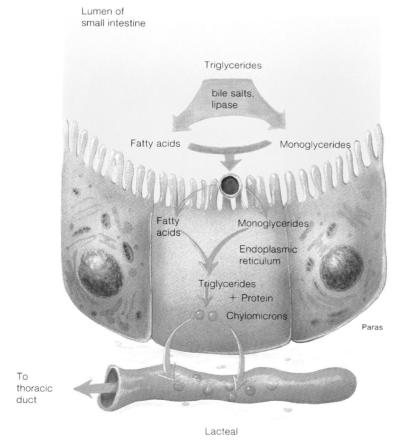

Absorption of Fatty Acids and Monoglycerides from Micelles
Figure 26.44

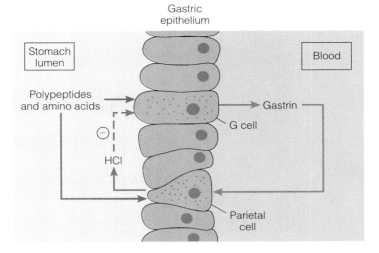

Stimulation of Gastric Acid (HCl) Secretion
Figure 26.45

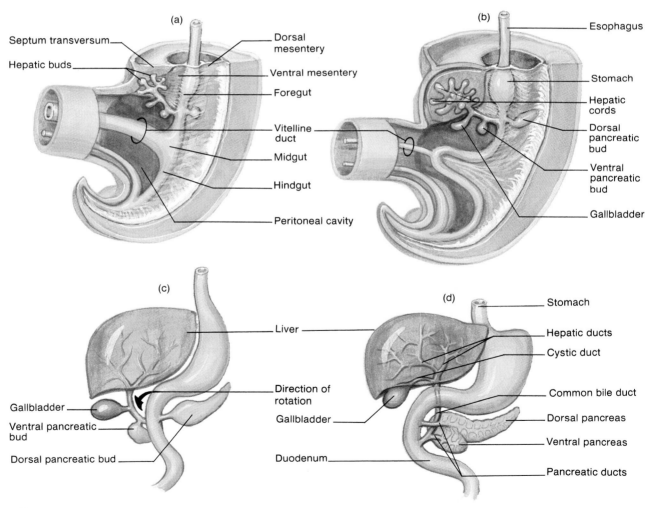

Waldrop

Development of Digestive System
Box Figure 26.1, Figure 1

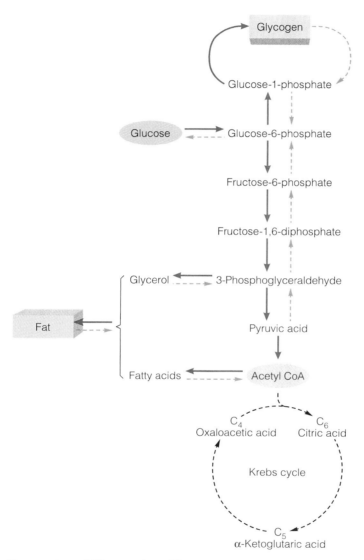

Conversion of Glucose into Glycogen
Figure 27.2

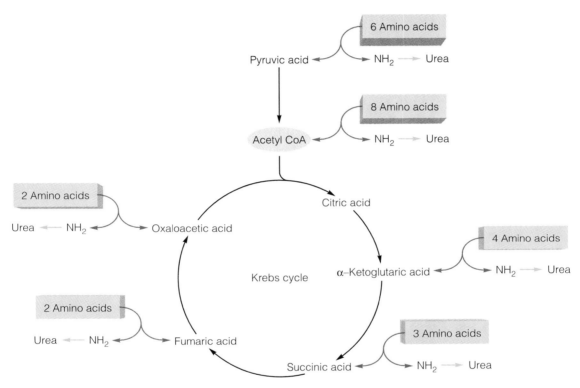

Pathways by which Amino Acids can be Catabolized for Energy
Figure 27.6

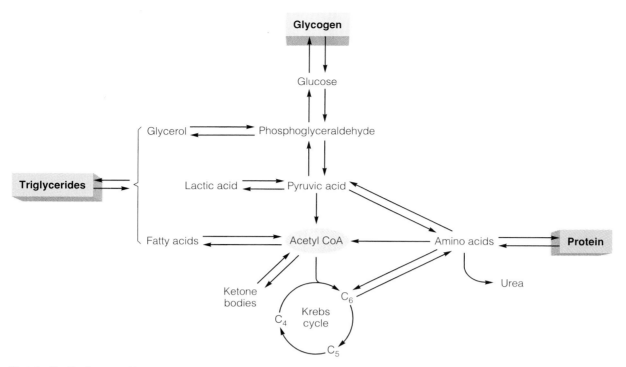

Metabolic Pathways Showing how Glycogen, Fat, and Protein can be Interconverted
Figure 27.7

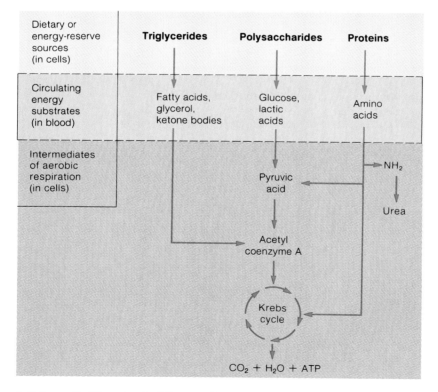

A Schematic Flowchart of Energy Pathways in the Body
Figure 27.8

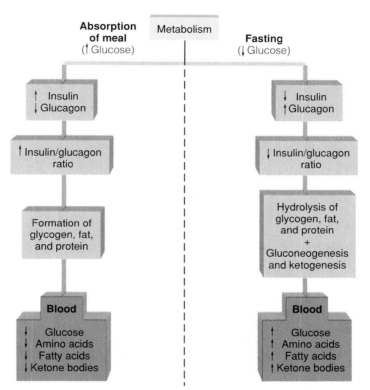

Inverse Relationship between Insulin and Glucagon during Absorption and Fasting
Figure 27.16

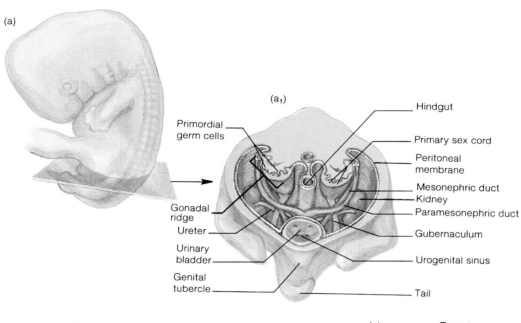

(a)

(a₁)

Primordial germ cells

Hindgut

Primary sex cord

Peritoneal membrane

Mesonephric duct

Kidney

Paramesonephric duct

Gubernaculum

Gonadal ridge

Ureter

Urinary bladder

Genital tubercle

Urogenital sinus

Tail

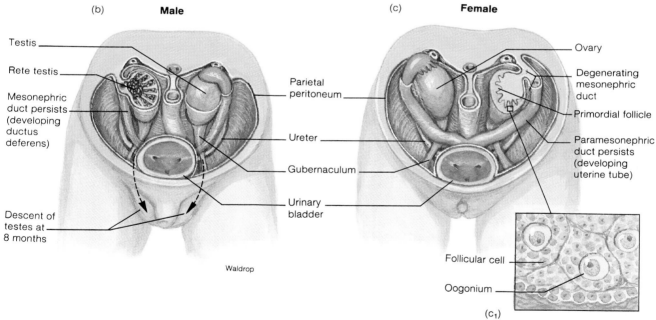

(b) **Male**

Testis

Rete testis

Mesonephric duct persists (developing ductus deferens)

Descent of testes at 8 months

Parietal peritoneum

Ureter

Gubernaculum

Urinary bladder

Waldrop

(c) **Female**

Ovary

Degenerating mesonephric duct

Primordial follicle

Paramesonephric duct persists (developing uterine tube)

Follicular cell

Oogonium

(c₁)

Differentiation of Male and Female Gonads
Box Figure 28.1, Figure 1

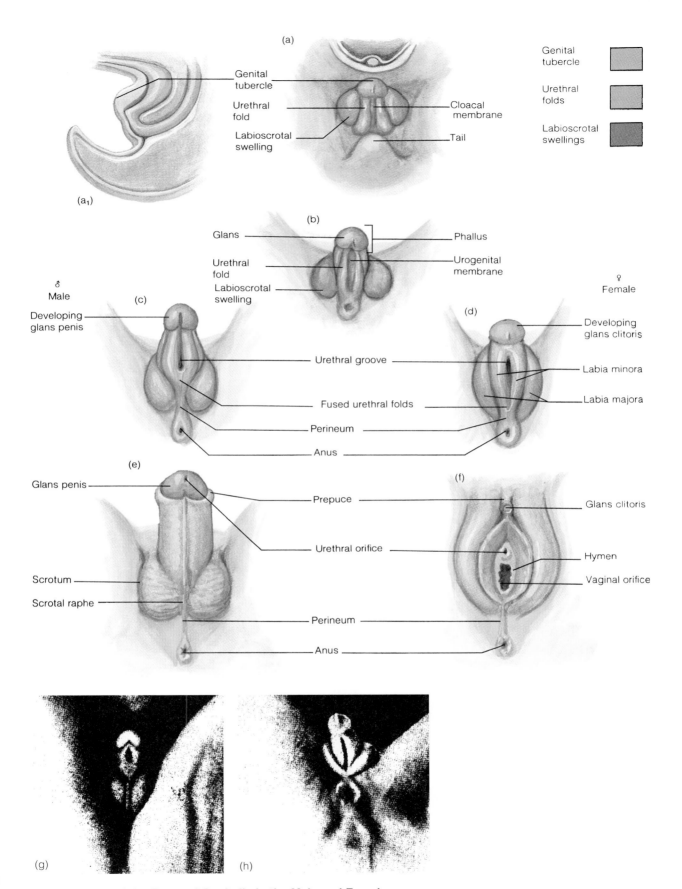

Differentiation of the External Genitalia in the Male and Female
Box Figure 28.1, Figure 2

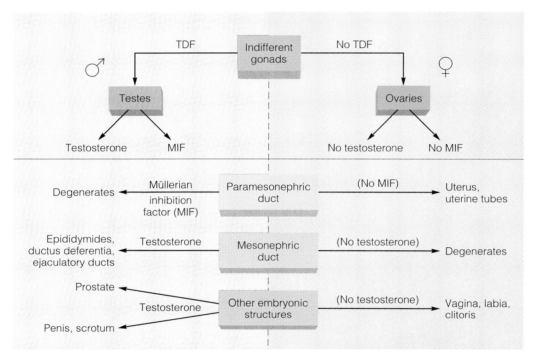

Development of the Male and Female Accessory Sex Organs and Genitalia
Box Figure 28.1, Figure 3

(a)

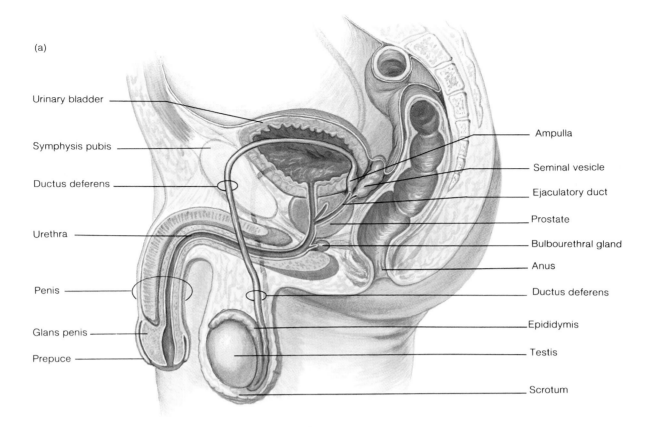

Urinary bladder

Symphysis pubis

Ductus deferens

Urethra

Penis

Glans penis

Prepuce

Ampulla

Seminal vesicle

Ejaculatory duct

Prostate

Bulbourethral gland

Anus

Ductus deferens

Epididymis

Testis

Scrotum

(b)

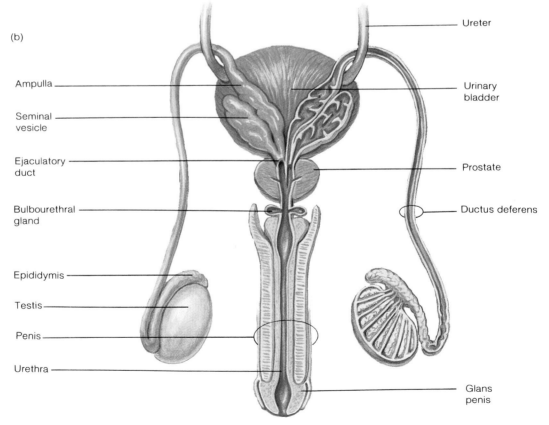

Ureter

Ampulla

Seminal vesicle

Ejaculatory duct

Bulbourethral gland

Epididymis

Testis

Penis

Urethra

Urinary bladder

Prostate

Ductus deferens

Glans penis

Basic Anatomy of Male Reproductive System
Figure 28.7

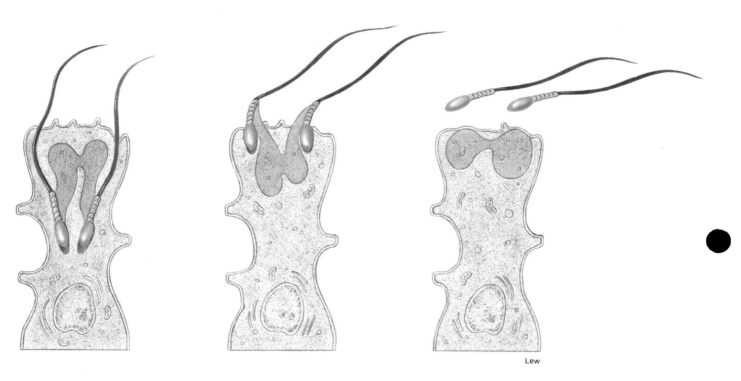

Formation of Spermatozoa
Figure 28.14

Lew

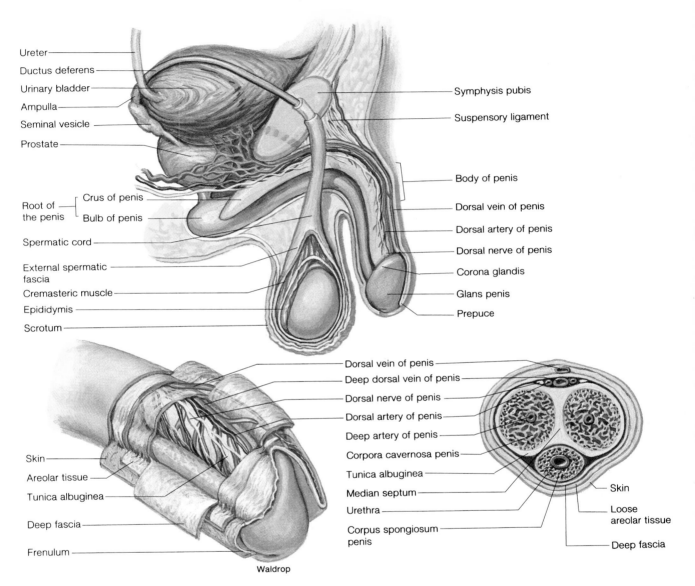

Ureter

Ductus deferens

Urinary bladder

Ampulla

Seminal vesicle

Prostate

Root of the penis ⎡ Crus of penis ⎣ Bulb of penis

Spermatic cord

External spermatic fascia

Cremasteric muscle

Epididymis

Scrotum

Symphysis pubis

Suspensory ligament

Body of penis

Dorsal vein of penis

Dorsal artery of penis

Dorsal nerve of penis

Corona glandis

Glans penis

Prepuce

Skin

Areolar tissue

Tunica albuginea

Deep fascia

Frenulum

Dorsal vein of penis

Deep dorsal vein of penis

Dorsal nerve of penis

Dorsal artery of penis

Deep artery of penis

Corpora cavernosa penis

Tunica albuginea

Median septum

Urethra

Corpus spongiosum penis

Skin

Loose areolar tissue

Deep fascia

Waldrop

Structure of the Penis
Figure 28.22

171

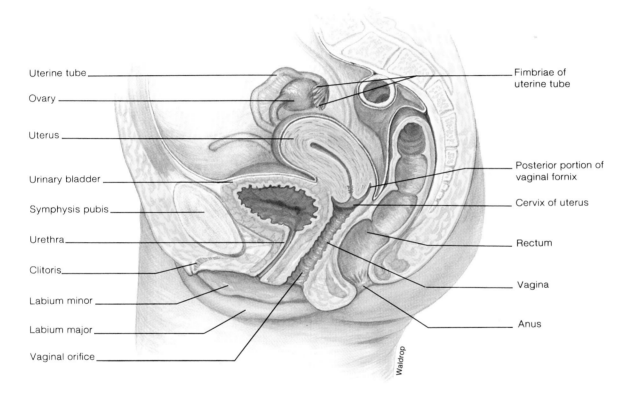

Organs of the Female Reproductive System in Sagittal View
Figure 29.1

Uterine tube

Ovary

Uterus

Urinary bladder

Symphysis pubis

Urethra

Clitoris

Labium minor

Labium major

Vaginal orifice

Fimbriae of
uterine tube

Posterior portion of
vaginal fornix

Cervix of uterus

Rectum

Vagina

Anus

Waldrop

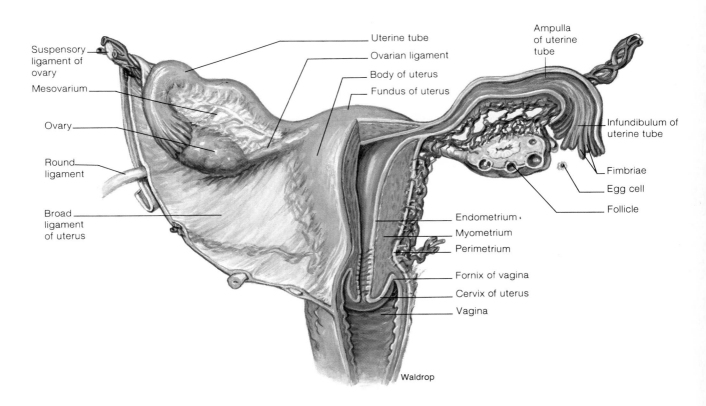

Suspensory ligament of ovary

Mesovarium

Ovary

Round ligament

Broad ligament of uterus

Uterine tube

Ovarian ligament

Body of uterus

Fundus of uterus

Ampulla of uterine tube

Infundibulum of uterine tube

Fimbriae

Egg cell

Follicle

Endometrium

Myometrium

Perimetrium

Fornix of vagina

Cervix of uterus

Vagina

Waldrop

Basic Anatomy of Female Reproductive System in Anterior View
Figure 29.4

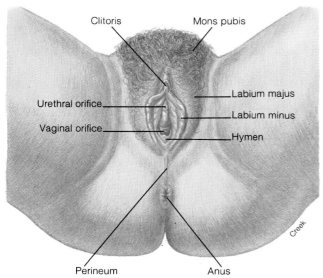

Clitoris

Mons pubis

Urethral orifice

Labium majus

Labium minus

Vaginal orifice

Hymen

Creek

Perineum

Anus

External Female Genitalia
Figure 29.7

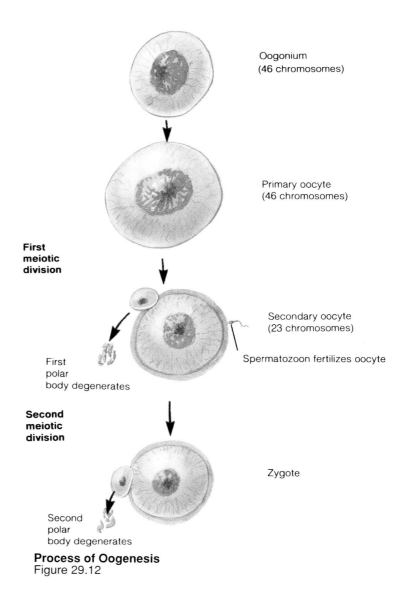

Oogonium
(46 chromosomes)

Primary oocyte
(46 chromosomes)

**First
meiotic
division**

Secondary oocyte
(23 chromosomes)

First
polar
body degenerates

Spermatozoon fertilizes oocyte

**Second
meiotic
division**

Zygote

Second
polar
body degenerates

Process of Oogenesis
Figure 29.12

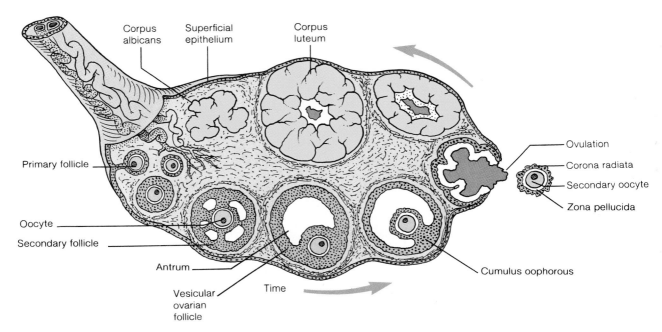

Ovary and Stages of Ovum and Follicle Development
Figure 29.13

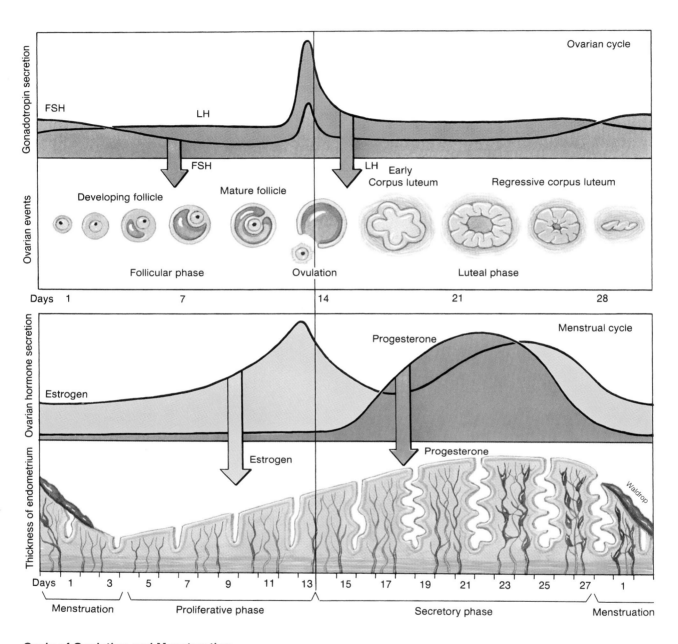

Cycle of Ovulation and Menstruation
Figure 29.14

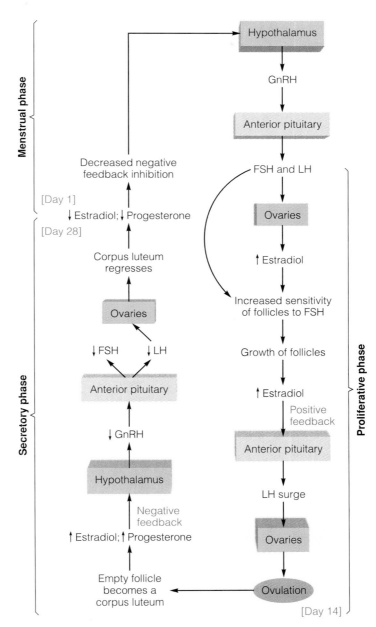

Endocrine Control of the Ovarian and Menstrual Cycles
Figure 29.16

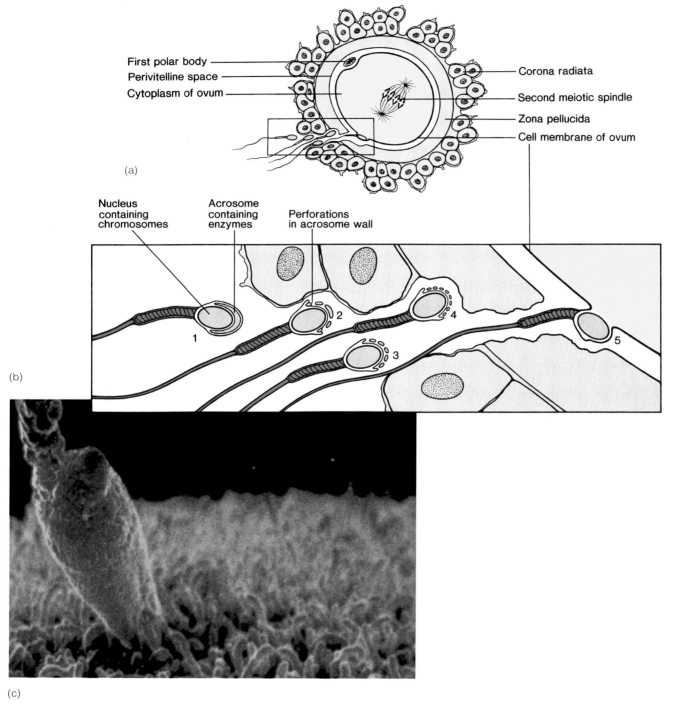

(a)

First polar body
Perivitelline space
Cytoplasm of ovum

Corona radiata
Second meiotic spindle
Zona pellucida
Cell membrane of ovum

Nucleus
containing
chromosomes

Acrosome
containing
enzymes

Perforations
in acrosome wall

(b)

1
2
3
4
5

(c)

Process of Fertilization
Figure 30.1

178

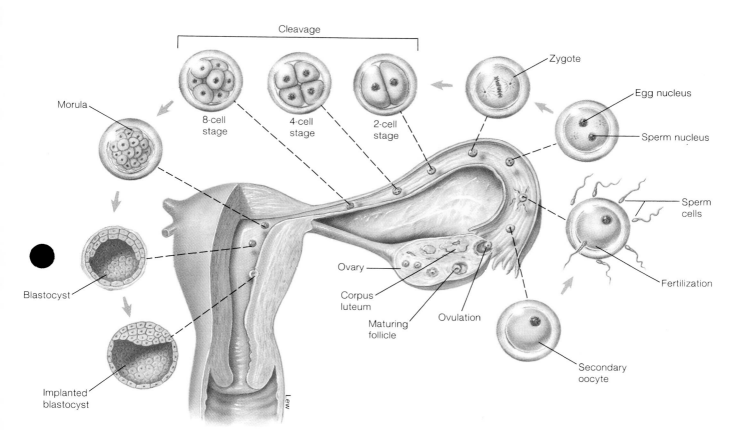

Cleavage

Zygote

Egg nucleus

Morula

8-cell stage

4-cell stage

2-cell stage

Sperm nucleus

Sperm cells

Blastocyst

Ovary

Corpus luteum

Maturing follicle

Ovulation

Fertilization

Implanted blastocyst

Secondary oocyte

Lew

Ovarian Cycle and Fertilization
Figure 30.6

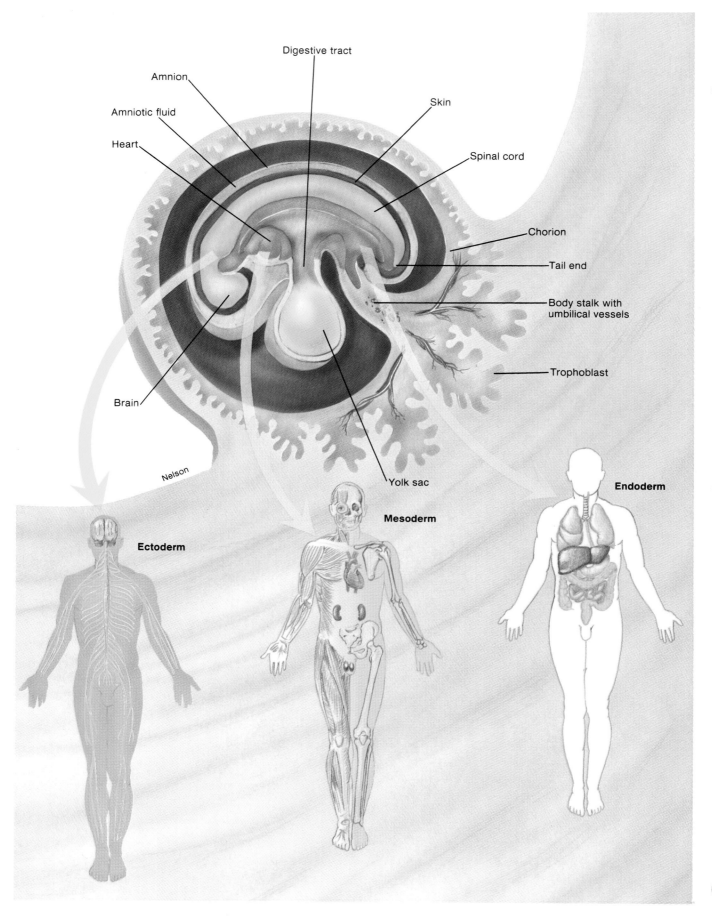

Body Systems Developed from Primary Germ Layers
Figure 30.10

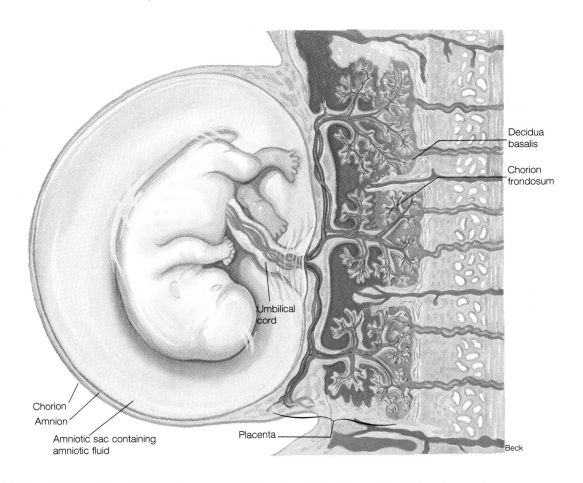

Embryo, Extraembryonic Membranes, and Placenta at about 7 weeks of Development
Figure 30.13

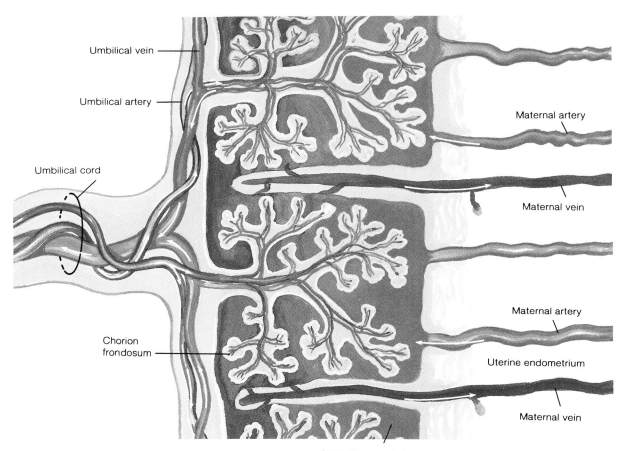

Umbilical vein

Umbilical artery

Umbilical cord

Chorion frondosum

Maternal artery

Maternal vein

Maternal artery

Uterine endometrium

Maternal vein

Intervillous pool of maternal blood

Circulation of Blood within the Placenta
Figure 30.15

Line Art

Fig. 12.1 From John W. Hole, Jr., *Human Anatomy and Physiology,* 6th ed. Copyright © 1993 Wm. C. Brown Communications, Inc., Dubuque, Iowa. All Rights Reserved. Reprinted by permission.

Fig. 15.1 From John W. Hole, Jr., and Karen A. Koos, *Human Anatomy,* 2d ed. Copyright © 1994 Wm. C. Brown Communications, Inc., Dubuque, Iowa. All Rights Reserved. Reprinted by permission.

Fig. 15.7 From John W. Hole, Jr., *Human Anatomy and Physiology,* 6th edition. Copyright © 1993 Wm. C. Brown Communications, Inc., Dubuque, Iowa. All Rights Reserved. Reprinted by permission.

Fig. 15.19 From Joan G. Creagher, *Human Anatomy and Physiology,* 2d ed. Copyright © Wm. C. Brown Communications, Inc., Dubuque, Iowa. All Rights Reserved. Reprinted by permission.

Fig. 15.22 From John W. Hole, Jr., *Human Anatomy and Physiology,* 6th ed. Copyright © 1993 Wm. C. Brown Communications, Inc., Dubuque, Iowa. All Rights Reserved. Reprinted by permission.

Fig. 15.24 From Joan G. Creagher, *Human Anatomy and Physiology,* 2d ed. Copyright © Wm. C. Brown Communications, Inc., Dubuque, Iowa. All Rights Reserved. Reprinted by permission.

Fig. 18.19 From John W. Hole, Jr., *Human Anatomy and Physiology,* 6th ed. Copyright © 1993 Wm. C. Brown Communications, Inc., Dubuque, Iowa. All Rights Reserved. Reprinted by permission.

Fig. 18.28 From John W. Hole, Jr., *Human Anatomy and Physiology,* 6th ed. Copyright © 1993 Wm. C. Brown Communications, Inc., Dubuque, Iowa. All Rights Reserved. Reprinted by permission.

Fig. 20.4 From John W. Hole, Jr., *Human Anatomy and Physiology,* 6th ed. Copyright © 1993 Wm. C. Brown Communications, Inc., Dubuque, Iowa. All Rights Reserved. Reprinted by permission.

Fig. 20.8 Adapted from A. Marchand, "Case of the Month, Circulating Anticoagulants: Chasing the Diagnosis," in *Diagnostic Medicine,* June 1983, p. 14. Used by permission.

Fig. 21.3 From John W. Hole, Jr., *Human Anatomy and Physiology,* 5th ed. Copyright © 1990 Wm. C. Brown Communications, Inc. Dubuque, Iowa. All Rights Reserved. Reprinted by permission.

Fig. 21.21a From John W. Hole, Jr., *Human Anatomy and Physiology,* 6th ed. Copyright © 1993 Wm. C. Brown Communications, Inc., Dubuque, Iowa. All Rights Reserved. Reprinted by permission.

Fig. 21.31 From John W. Hole, Jr., *Human Anatomy and Physiology,* 6th ed. Copyright © 1993 Wm. C. Brown Communications, Inc., Dubuque, Iowa. All Rights Reserved. Reprinted by permission.

Fig. 22.6 Source: Data from Bjorn Folkow and Eric Neil, *Circulation.* Copyright © 1971 Oxford University Press.

Fig. 22.17 Adapted from P. Astrand and K. Rodahl, *Textbook of Work Physiology,* 3d edition, copyright 1986 McGraw-Hill, Inc., New York. Used by permission of the author.

Fig. 24.22 From John W. Hole, Jr., *Human Anatomy and Physiology,* 6th ed. Copyright © 1993 Wm. C. Brown Communications, Inc., Dubuque, Iowa. All Rights Reserved. Reprinted by permission.

Fig. 25.3 From John W. Hole, Jr., *Human Anatomy and Physiology,* 6th edition. Copyright © 1993 Wm. C. Brown Communications, Inc., Dubuque, Iowa. All Rights Reserved. Reprinted by permission.

Fig. 25.6 From John W. Hole, Jr., *Human Anatomy and Physiology,* 6th ed. Copyright © 1993 Wm. C. Brown Communications, Inc., Dubuque, Iowa. All Rights Reserved. Reprinted by permission.

Fig. 26.7 From John W. Hole, Jr., *Human Anatomy and Physiology,* 6th ed. Copyright © 1993 Wm. C. Brown Communications, Inc., Dubuque, Iowa. All Rights Reserved. Reprinted by permission.

Fig. 26.12 From John W. Hole, Jr., *Human Anatomy and Physiology,* 6th ed. Copyright © 1993 Wm. C. Brown Communications, Inc., Dubuque, Iowa. All Rights Reserved. Reprinted by permission.

Fig. 26.17 From John W. Hole, Jr., *Human Anatomy and Physiology,* 6th ed. Copyright © 1993 Wm. C. Brown Communications, Inc., Dubuque, Iowa. All Rights Reserved. Reprinted by permission.

Fig. 26.30 From John W. Hole, Jr., *Human Anatomy and Physiology,* 6th ed. Copyright © 1993 Wm. C. Brown Communications, Inc., Dubuque, Iowa. All Rights Reserved. Reprinted by permission.

Fig. 28.7 From John W. Hole, Jr., *Human Anatomy and Physiology,* 6th ed. Copyright © 1993 Wm. C. Brown Communications, Inc., Dubuque, Iowa. All Rights Reserved. Reprinted by permission.

Fig. 29.1 From John W. Hole, Jr., *Human Anatomy and Physiology,* 6th ed. Copyright © 1993 Wm. C. Brown Communications, Inc., Dubuque, Iowa. All Rights Reserved. Reprinted by permission.

Fig. 29.14 From John W. Hole, Jr., *Human Anatomy and Physiology,* 6th ed. Copyright © 1993 Wm. C. Brown Communications, Inc., Dubuque, Iowa. All Rights Reserved. Reprinted by permission.

Photos

Fig. 1.11 © Dr. Sheril Burton

Fig. 3.30 a-2 thru e-2 © Edwin A. Reschke

Table 7.2 © Edwin A. Reschke/Peter Arnold, Inc.

Box Fig. 8.1, Fig. 2 Ted Conde

Fig. 12.2b © Edwin A. Reschke

Fig. 12.5b © John D. Cunningham/Visuals Unlimited

Fig. 12.10a © Dr. H. E. Huxley

Fig. 15.3a,b and c Kent M. Van De Graaff

Fig. 15.24b © Per Kjeldsen, University of Michigan, Ann Arbor

Fig. 18.18 Kent M. Van De Graaff

Fig. 18.37 © Per Kjeldsen, University of Michigan, Ann Arbor

Fig. 19.1b © Edwin A. Reschke

Fig. 21.21b From: Practische Intleekunde from J. Dankmeyer, H. G. Lambers, and J. M. F. Landsmearr. Bohn, Scheltma and Holkema

Fig. 26.31c © Victor B. Eichler, Ph.D.

Fig. 26.38 © Edwin A. Reschke

Box Fig. 28.1, Fig. 2 © Dr. Landrum Shettles

Box Fig. 28.1, Fig. 3 © Dr. Landrum Shettles

Fig. 30.1c © David Phillips/Visuals Unlimited